BIPOLAR DEPRESSION

A Comprehensive Guide

BIPOLAR DEPRESSION

A Comprehensive Guide

Edited by

Rif S. El-Mallakh, M.D.

S. Nassir Ghaemi, M.D., M.P.H.

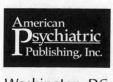

American Psychiatric Publishing, Inc.

Washington, DC
London, England

To buy 25–99 copies of any APPI title at a 20% discount, please contact APPI Customer Service at appi@psych.org or 800-368-5777. To buy 100 or more copies of the same title, please e-mail bulksales@psych.org for a price quote

Copyright © 2006 American Psychiatric Publishing, Inc.
ALL RIGHTS RESERVED

Manufactured in the United States of America on acid-free paper
10   09   08   07   06   5   4   3   2   1
First Edition

Typeset in Adobe's Palatino and Christiana

American Psychiatric Publishing, Inc.
1000 Wilson Boulevard
Arlington, VA 22209-3901
www.appi.org

Library of Congress Cataloging-in-Publication Data
Bipolar depression : a comprehensive guide / edited by Rif S. El-Mallakh,
    S. Nassir Ghaemi. — 1st ed.
        p. ; cm.
    Includes bibliographical references and index.
    ISBN 1-58562-171-4 (pbk. : alk. paper)
    1. Manic-depressive illness.   I. El-Mallakh, Rif S., 1956– .
    II. Ghaemi, S. Nassir.
    [DNLM: 1. Bipolar Disorder.   WM 207 B6153 2006]
    RC516.B515 2006
    616.89′5—dc22   2006001944

British Library Cataloguing in Publication Data
A CIP record is available from the British Library.

CONTENTS

CONTRIBUTORS

Julia Appelbaum, M.D.
Stanley Research Center, Division of Psychiatry, Faculty of Health Sciences, Ben Gurion University of the Negev, Beer Sheva, Israel

Robert H. Belmaker, M.D.
Professor of Psychiatry, Faculty of Health Sciences, Ben Gurion University of the Negev, Beer Sheva, Israel

Polina Eidelman, B.A.
Graduate Student, Massachusetts General Hospital, Boston, Massachusetts

Rif S. El-Mallakh, M.D.
Director, Mood Disorders Research Program; Associate Professor, Department of Psychiatry and Behavioral Sciences, University of Louisville School of Medicine, Louisville, Kentucky

S. Nassir Ghaemi, M.D., M.P.H.
Associate Professor, Department of Psychiatry and Behavioral Sciences, Rollins School of Public Health; Director, Bipolar Disorder Research Program, Emory University, Atlanta, Georgia

Frederick K. Goodwin, M.D.
Center for Neuroscience, Medical Progress, and Society; Psychopharmacology Research Center; Research Professor, Department of Psychiatry and Behavioral Sciences, George Washington University, Washington, D.C.

Elizabeth P. Hayden, Ph.D.
Assistant Professor, Department of Psychology, University of Western Ontario, London, Ontario, Canada

Anoop Karippot, M.D.
Assistant Professor, Division of Child and Adolescent Psychiatry, Bingham Child Guidance Center, University of Louisville School of Medicine, Louisville, Kentucky

Joseph Levine, M.D.
Associate Professor of Psychiatry, Stanley Research Center, Division of Psychiatry, Faculty of Health Sciences, Ben Gurion University of the Negev, Beer Sheva, Israel

John I. Nurnberger Jr., M.D., Ph.D.
Joyce and Iver Small Professor of Psychiatry, Professor of Medical and Molecular Genetics, Institute of Psychiatric Research, Indiana University School of Medicine, Indianapolis, Indiana

Michael J. Ostacher, M.D., M.P.H.
Associate Medical Director, Bipolar Clinic and Research Program, Massachusetts General Hospital; Instructor, Harvard Medical School, Boston, Massachusetts

Jaclyn Saggese, B.A.
Center for Neuroscience, Medical Progress, and Society; Psychopharmacology Research Center; Department of Psychiatry and Behavioral Sciences, George Washington University, Washington, D.C.

Alan C. Swann, M.D.
Pat R. Rutherford Jr. Professor and Vice Chair of Research, Department of Psychiatry and Behavioral Sciences, University of Texas Medical School, Houston, Texas

Francesc Colom, Psy.D., M.Sc., Ph.D.
Head of Psychoeducation and Psychological Treatment Areas, Bipolar Disorders Program, Stanley Research Center, University of Barcelona, Barcelona, Spain

Eduard Vieta, M.D.
Director of the Bipolar Disorders Program, Stanley Research Center, University of Barcelona, Barcelona, Spain

DIAGNOSIS OF
BIPOLAR DEPRESSION

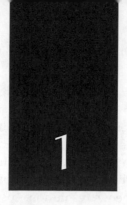

DIAGNOSIS OF BIPOLAR DEPRESSION

S. Nassir Ghaemi, M.D., M.P.H.
Jaclyn Saggese, B.A.
Frederick K. Goodwin, M.D.

ALTHOUGH DEPRESSION IS the most common presentation of bipolar disorder, a history of mania or hypomania is required for its diagnosis. Identifying these two behaviors defines the diagnostic problem that bipolar depression represents: when faced with a depressed patient, it can be extremely difficult for the clinician to validate the depression as stemming from bipolar disorder.

Generally speaking, determining that a patient currently meets criteria for a major depressive episode is straightforward. What is not straightforward, and therefore demands attention, is determining whether the patient's history is consistent with unipolar or bipolar depression. We suggest here a hierarchical model for such a diagnostic assessment, based on the validators of diagnosis used in psychiatric nosology.

THE VALIDATORS OF DIAGNOSIS

The classic validators of psychiatric diagnoses were first discussed by Eli Robins and Samuel Guze in 1970 in reference to schizophrenia. They identified five validators: signs and symptoms, delimitation from other disorders, the follow-up study (outcome), family history, and laboratory tests. The basic rationale for having multiple validators for a psychiatric diagnosis is the absence of a "gold standard." Whereas in medicine clinicians often argue over a potential diagnosis only to have the pathologist declare the right answer, in psychiatry there is no such definitive and instantaneous resolution—psychiatry has no pathologist. (In fact, since many pathologists spent entire careers searching in vain for simple brain abnormalities in patients with schizophrenia, it had become something of a rueful joke to say that schizophrenia is the "graveyard of pathologists.") In the absence of a specimen from an organ, psychiatric nosologists like Robins and Guze returned to the classic work of Emil Kraepelin, who, noting the failures of neuropathology to reveal the causes of mental illness, emphasized that "diagnosis is prognosis" (Ghaemi 2003), by which he meant that a psychiatric diagnosis is most clearly established by assessing the longitudinal course of illness.

This perspective contrasts with the psychoanalytic tradition developed in the United States and, to some extent, with the focus on phenomenology as it developed among some European scholars, such as Kurt Schneider (Janzarik 1998), for whom diagnosis was based substantially on the assessment of the patients' current symptoms (Ghaemi 2003). Kraepelin's approach argues that cross-sectional symptoms, no matter how well understood, are inadequate for diagnosing a disorder and that the course of illness is just as important, if not more so.

Robins and Guze added the Kraepelinian criterion of course to the standard symptom-oriented approach to diagnosis in the United States. They further added the criteria of family history, in order to incorporate the influence of genetics, and laboratory tests, in the hopes for more objective measures of illness. Since diagnostically useful laboratory tests have not been developed, over time, that criterion was replaced in practice by a weaker, yet still sometimes serviceable, alternative: treatment response. Actually, we would suggest that treatment *nonresponse* is a stronger diagnostic validator than treatment response because it has become clear over the last few decades that psychotropic (and other) medications are largely nonspecific. The neo-Kraepelinian paradigm that Robins and Guze put forward quickly led to the revolution in psychiatric nosology that resulted in DSM-III (in 1980), partly because it seemed that Kraepelin's diagnostic categories were finally therapeutically useful (Ghaemi 2003). We knew that lithium treated mania, tricyclic antidepressants treated depression, and phenothiazines treated schizophrenia, yet experience and research taught us that lithium can also treat depression, phenothiazines can treat mania, and antidepressants can treat many other conditions (including bipolar depression, depressive symptoms in schizophrenia, and anxiety disorders). Therefore, looking at treatment nonresponse may lead to more specific results: antidepressant nonresponse raises the suspicion of nonunipolar depression (Ghaemi et al. 2004b), antipsychotics alone are largely ineffective in depression (Dube et al. 2002; Tohen et al. 2003), and lithium is mostly ineffective in schizophrenia (Leucht et al. 2003).

Today, the original validators of diagnosis are generally conceptualized as only four: phenomenology, course of illness, genetics, and treatment nonresponse. The assessment of bipolar depression is best organized around these four validators.

PHENOMENOLOGY

At a superficial level, the phenomenology of bipolar depression can be described as twofold: past mania (or hypomania) and current depression.

The diagnosis of past manic or hypomanic episodes is where the standard DSM-IV-TR–based approach to bipolar depression begins and ends. This is a necessary but insufficient approach to diagnosing bipolar depression. While the presence of past manic or hypomanic episodes in the depressed patients meets the diagnostic criteria for bipolar depression, the apparent absence of such episodes does not adequately rule out bipolar depression. There are at least two reasons for this: First, type I or type II bipolar disorder may still be present in the absence of the patient's report of past manic/hypomanic episodes simply because the patient may not be adequately reporting past manic symptoms. Research shows that about half of patients with manic episodes have been shown to lack insight into their manic symptoms (Ghaemi and Rosenquist 2004; Ghaemi et al. 1995). It is important to interview family members, who are known to report their relatives' mania twice as frequently as the patients themselves (Keitner et al. 1996) (other factors like faulty memory for past events while acutely depressed are also relevant). Therefore, reliance on the patient's self-report, even with the most sophisticated clinical interviewer, will lead to underdiagnosis of bipolar disorder. Second, DSM-IV-TR is not the last word in the nosology of bipolar disorder. It may turn out that broader definitions may be valid. In other words, as Kraepelin suggested, nosological research may validate the diagnosis of bipolar illness without the presence of manic or hypomanic episodes (Kraepelin 1921).

Nonetheless, it is useful to begin with the issue of how one identifies past manic or hypomanic episodes. Besides talking to family members and getting outside sources of information, clinicians should also be wary of their own tendency to engage in what social psychologists call "diagnosis by prototype" (Cantor et al. 1980; Westen and Shedler 2000). In medicine, this is both the benefit and bane of having working experience: over time, one sees many patients with a certain diagnosis who resemble each other in certain traits, such as how they talk, how they dress, or their nonverbal behavior. Within minutes, experienced clinicians begin to form intuitive hunches about the patient's diagnosis or symptoms. Often these hunches are proven right, but if they are not followed up with more systematic assessments, clinicians may get caught in a vicious cycle of their own self-fulfilling habits: they will see certain patients as having certain diagnoses, and rarely can they be proven right or wrong. Yet patients can be depressed, and not appear depressed; they can be even psychotic, and not seem psychotic; and, in the case of bipolar disorder, they can be fully manic, and not appear manic at all, especially if one possesses a mental prototype in which manic patients must be euphoric, grandiosely psychotic, and bizarre.

The assessment of manic symptoms should not be simply intuitive and impressionistic, as is often the case in actual clinical practice. Like depression, where one focuses on certain neurovegetative symptoms, clinicians should carefully assess the cardinal symptoms of mania. Yet many clinicians do not even clearly understand what those cardinal symptoms are (Sprock 1988). Just as "SIGECAPS" (originally developed by Dr. Carey Gross at Massachusetts General Hospital [MGH]) has proven useful as a mnemonic for depression, "DIGFAST" (originally developed by Dr. William Falk at MGH), in our opinion, is as an important mnemonic to force clinicians to systematically assess manic symptoms.

DIGFAST: A Mnemonic for Mania

DIGFAST is a mnemonic aid for the following concepts:

Distractibility—An inability to maintain one's concentration, as opposed to the decreased concentration of depression, where one is unable to initiate concentration. In mania, this leads to the initiation of multiple tasks, none of which are finished.

Insomnia—A decreased *need* for sleep, as opposed to the decreased sleep of depressive insomnia. The patient sleeps less, but has intact or increased energy the next day. Alternatively, there is no change in amount of sleep, but the patient's energy level is increased.

Grandiosity—Inflated self-esteem; it need not involve delusions.

Flight of ideas—A subjective experience of racing thoughts.

Activities—An increase in goal-directed activities (social, sexual, school, work, and home).

Speech—Pressured; an objective sign. A subjective alternative is increased talkativeness, determined by asking whether the patient has been more talkative than when euthymic.

Thoughtlessness—Commonly called *risk-taking behavior*—an increase in pleasurable activities with the potential for painful consequences. Four such behaviors that should be routinely assessed are sexual indiscretions, spending sprees, impulsive traveling, and reckless driving.

Mania is diagnosed when euphoric mood is present for one week with three of the DIGFAST symptoms, or irritable mood with four symptoms, and there is significant social or occupational dysfunction. If functioning is unimpaired, and manic symptoms last at least 4 days, hypomania is diagnosed. If symptoms last less than 4 days, bipolar disorder not otherwise specified is diagnosed.

Strict reliance on euphoria grossly underestimates the behaviors in bipolar illness, since irritability alone is sufficient as the primary mood change in mania, and since mixed episodes (where mood is depressed) are almost as common as pure manic episodes (Goodwin and Jamison 1990). Irritability, expressed as anger attacks, is more common in bipolar than in unipolar depression (Perlis et al. 2004), and its occurrence should trigger careful assessment of DIGFAST criteria. Other DIGFAST triggers are the depressive features of bipolar illness noted below.

According to DSM-IV-TR criteria, hypomania is distinguished from mania on the basis of social or occupational dysfunction, not specific manic symptoms. Since patients often underestimate interpersonal dysfunction, family reports become essential. Therefore, it is difficult, if not impossible, to rule out bipolar disorder without family or another third-person report.

Beyond DSM–IV–TR

If past manic or hypomanic episodes are not present or if the history of these episodes is confusing and they cannot be definitively ruled in or out, then we would recommend that clinicians move on to assessing the likelihood of bipolar illness using the four validators of psychiatric diagnosis, beginning with an assessment of depressive phenomenology, followed by course of illness, genetics, and, lastly, treatment nonresponse. None of the following concepts are to be found in DSM-IV-TR,

TABLE 1–1.   Differences in phenomenology between bipolar and unipolar depression

More common in bipolar than in unipolar depression:
  Atypical symptoms
  Psychosis
  Depressive mixed state
  Anxious/agitated depression
  Anergic depression*
  Irritability/anger attacks*

*Suspected, but uncertain.

which again, we emphasize, should be seen as a step in the nosological history of bipolar disorder, not the end of that history. Thus, the other validators of diagnosis should be seen as just as relevant as the single validator employed in DSM-IV-TR (i.e., presence or absence of past manic or hypomanic episodes).

Depressive Phenomenology

The current symptoms of bipolar depression have been thought by many to be similar to those seen in unipolar depression. Yet it appears that there are differences between unipolar and bipolar in the phenomenological presentation of depression. These likely differences are highlighted in Table 1–1.

Atypical depressive symptoms seem to be more common in bipolar than in unipolar depression (Agosti and Stewart, 2001; Benazzi 1999, 2001a; Ghaemi et al. 2002; Mitchell et al. 2001). In the National Institutes of Mental Health Collaborative Depression Study, a 20-year, prospective cohort study of depressed patients, atypical depressive features were a predictor of bipolar disorder, as opposed to unipolar depression (Akiskal et al. 1995). DSM-IV-TR criteria for atypical features include increased sleep, increased appetite, rejection sensitivity, leaden paralysis, and mood reactivity. The DSM-IV-TR definition of atypical depression is stricter than some clinical definitions, which focus mainly on the sleep and appetite features. An interesting clinical observation is that most bipolar patients have only one of the reversed neurovegetative symptoms; that is, many patients experience increased sleep but decreased appetite, or vice versa. If one defines typical depression as decreased sleep and appetite, and atypical depression as the presence of any of the atypical features noted above, then about 90% of bipolar depressive episodes involve atypical features, in contrast to only about half of unipolar depressive episodes (Ghaemi et al. 2004a).

Psychotic depression also appears to be more common in bipolar depression than in unipolar depression (Mitchell et al. 1992, 2001; Parker et al. 2000). Often the presence of psychotic symptoms can be difficult to establish. This may be because psychotic depressed patients seem to have more insight into their symptoms than do manic or schizophrenic patients and thus are more likely to hide these symptoms (Dell'Osso et al. 2002). Depressive symptoms that may be more prominent in such psychotic depressed patients, compared with nonpsychotic depressed patients, include markedly increased guilt and psychomotor agitation or retardation (Schatzberg and Rothschild 1992). Thus, in the guarded, very agitated, guilty bipolar depressed patient, one should have a high index of suspicion for concomitant psychosis. Clinical experience also suggests that psychotic depression in a young person is a common initial presentation of a bipolar illness. In such a person, especially if he or she has a family history of bipolar disorder, careful consideration should be given to the initial use of mood stabilizers, rather than antidepressants.

The depressive "mixed state" represents both major depression with manic symptoms that are subthreshold for the DSM-IV-TR definition of a mixed episode (Perugi et al. 1997). This presentation is similar, though not identical, to agitated depression (Akiskal et al. 2005), because most definitions of the depressive mixed state require the presence of two or three manic-like symptoms along with the major depressive episode (Benazzi 2004b). These manic-like symptoms are most frequently increased psychomotor activity, racing or crowded thoughts, and periods of decreased need for sleep. A number of studies have shown that such definitions of a depressive mixed state are quite common in bipolar type II depression in particular (Benazzi 2004a, 2004b) and much more common in bipolar illness than unipolar depression (Akiskal et al. 2000; Benazzi 2001b; Sato et al. 2003). In one report, Benazzi (2001b) found that depression with two manic-like symptoms was present in 71.8% of bipolar II patients versus 41.5% of unipolar patients, while depression with three such symptoms was present in 46.6% of bipolar II patients versus 7.6% of unipolar patients. In a follow-up study of 563 patients, Benazzi confirmed the prevalence of depressive mixed state, defined by the presence of three manic-like symptoms, as occurring in 49.5% of patients with bipolar disorder type II (Benazzi 2004b). (It is important to note that these reports may conflate hyperactivity and agitation.)

Outside of psychomotor agitated depression, there is also the question of whether anxious depression is related to bipolar disorder. The presence of anxiety along with the major depressive episode is a common occurrence. It is not generally considered diagnostically informative, though often such patients will have manic symptoms that can represent a depressive mixed state. The interesting clinical question is whether anxious depression, in the absence of other manic-like symptoms, is more common in bipolar than unipolar depression. Anxiety symptoms are extremely common in bipolar disorder, so that when the diagnostic criteria for anxiety are applied, lifetime comorbidity ranges from 55% to 90% (Boylan et al. 2004); consequently, comorbidity with anxiety has been reported to be more frequent than with unipolar depression. On the basis of extensive clinical experience, Koukopoulos and Koukopoulos (1999) suggest a link between anxiety and bipolar disorder, as does Perugi (Perugi and Akiskal 2002; Perugi et al. 1999). In perhaps the principal study for the diagnostic relevance of anxiety during depression, Benazzi et al. (2004) found that the presence of psychic tension and agitation was found in 15.4% of 336 persons with major depressive episodes (both unipolar and bipolar type II); this anxious tension predicted bipolar type II disorder in multivariate regression modeling.

It has frequently been reported that anergic depression is more commonly related to bipolar illness than to unipolar illness. This anergia partly represents the marked psychomotor retardation seen in melancholic depression. Although atypical and melancholic depression can be seen as contrasting (preserved mood reactivity in the former, marked anhedonia in the latter), some data suggest that they are both more frequent in bipolar than unipolar depression (Mitchell et al. 2001; Parker et al. 2000). To some extent, this possibility conflicts with the above hypothesis that anxious or agitated depression may reflect bipolarity. Indeed, some research suggests that psychomotor retardation may be more common in unipolar depression, although psychomotor agitation appears more frequently in bipolar depression (Mitchell et al. 1992). Although anergic depression is often identified with bipolar disorder, the extent of the literature supporting this view is rather limited, compared with the growing evidence that the depressive mixed state and variations of anxious and agitated depression may be more characteristic of bipolar than unipolar depression.

Irritability and anger attacks have also been linked to bipolar depression. Irritability can represent a component of the depressive mixed state, but, as with anxiety, the clinical question is whether irritability and anger during the major depressive episode (in the absence of other manic-like symptoms) are more characteristic of bipolar than unipolar illness. Benazzi and Akiskal (2005b) report that this is the case; they found that major depressive episodes with irritability were present in 59.7% of 348 patients with type II bipolar disorder versus 37.4% of

254 patients with unipolar depression. In a large unipolar sample, the prevalence of irritability with depression was also reported to be about 40% (Perlis et al. 2005). In 79 bipolar and unipolar subjects, anger attacks (which likely represent a subtype of marked irritability) were reported to be much more common in the bipolar (62%) than the unipolar group (26%) (Perlis et al. 2004). In sum, irritability per se, viewed as a separate symptom from other manic-like symptoms, may also be more common in bipolar than unipolar depression, but it should be noted that irritability can be difficult to define operationally and it may also be relatively nonspecific with respect to diagnosis.

In general, the phenomenology of major depression appears to differ between bipolar and unipolar depression. Atypical, psychotic, and depressive mixed state presentations seem to be rather well established as more common in bipolar than in unipolar. Anergic, melancholic, anxious, and irritable presentations may also prove to differ between the groups, though further research is needed to establish those associations.

Course of Illness

Differences also exist between bipolar and unipolar depression in the course of those conditions (Table 1–2). Kraepelin (1921) viewed the course of illness as the key diagnostic validator that differentiated illnesses. In the case of bipolar disorder, its earlier age at onset differentiates it from unipolar depression, which has a later age at onset range, with a median in the late 20s to early 30s. Follow-up studies of depressed patients with an age at onset below 25 or 30 indicate that such early-onset, depressed patients often develop bipolar disorder. In one study of 72 children who entered unipolar depression clinical trials at mean age of 12.3 years, 48.6% had developed manic or hypomanic episodes by the 10-year follow-up (Geller et al. 2001). In another study of 74 young adults (mean age 23.0 years) initially hospitalized for unipolar major depressive episodes, a similar number (46%) had developed manic or hypomanic episodes by the 15-year follow-up (Goldberg et al. 2001). In contrast, follow-up studies of samples with an initial mean age in the lower 30s report much lower rates of the manic switch to bipolar illness (12.5% in 559 patients followed for 11 years) (Akiskal et al. 1995).

It is important to realize that the most common first mood episode in bipolar disorder appears to be a major depressive episode, rather than a manic episode (Goodwin and Jamison 1990). Thus, as shown above, new-onset depression in a child or young adult has a high likelihood (estimated at about 50%) of becoming bipolar illness.

TABLE 1–2. Differences in course between bipolar and unipolar depression

More common in bipolar than in unipolar depression:
  Early age at onset
  Recurrence
  Postpartum
  Rapid cycling
  Brief duration of depressive episodes
  Baseline hyperthymic personality

Recurrence of mood episodes is much more common in bipolar than unipolar depression. About one quarter of patients with unipolar depression experienced no further mood episodes in a 13.5-year follow-up (Stephens and McHugh 1991), and those with a first major depressive episode are very likely to recover and be symptom free at the 12-year follow-up (Judd et al. 1998). In contrast, almost all bipolar patients experience a recurrent mood episode within 4 years of follow-up (Tohen et al. 1990), with the usual natural history averaging close to one mood episode per year (Kessing et al. 1998).

Postpartum onset of depressive episodes is likely more frequent in bipolar than unipolar depression (Freeman et al. 2001), though it is highly prevalent in both conditions. Rapid cycling (four or more episodes in a year) is highly uncommon in unipolar depression compared to bipolar disorder (Wolpert et al. 1990). This links to the observation that bipolar depressive episodes are briefer than unipolar depressive episodes. Although estimates differ among studies (Goodwin and Jamison 1990), the average untreated major depressive episode lasts 6–12 months in unipolar depression, versus 3–6 months in bipolar depression.

Baseline hyperthymic personality is another important course feature to assess (Cassano et al. 1992; Perugi et al. 2001). Obviously, when one is evaluating mood episodes, it is important to compare them to patients' baseline mood states, which, in effect, represent the usual personality of the patient. Hyperthymic personality is a state in which one is chronically hypomanic, with a personality that is bubbly, outgoing, and very extroverted. Typically, such persons need less sleep than most individuals (6 hours or less), and have a great deal of energy that they spend in work (workaholism) and social activities. They often also have a good deal of libido, and can have more interpersonal marital conflicts due to sexual indiscretions than the general population. Hyperthymic personality has been reported to be more frequent in families of persons with bipolar disorder (Chiaroni et al. 2004), and it is a predictor of antidepressant-induced mania (Henry et al. 2001b). Frequently, the diagnosis of bipolar disorder type II is difficult to make in patients with severe, recurrent, depressive episodes and hyperthymic personalities, rather than discrete, episodic, hypomanic episodes alternating with euthymic states.

Genetics

It is an often-underrecognized fact that the primary scientific basis for the distinction between bipolar and unipolar depression, as opposed to the broader concept of manic depressive illness, had to do with genetic studies. Classic research by Perris in the 1960s suggested that patients with bipolar disorder had family members that were diagnosable with bipolar disorder, whereas patients with unipolar depression had family members that were diagnosable with unipolar depression but not bipolar disorder (Perris 1966).

This literature on genetic studies has significant clinical relevance: if an individual with pure, unipolar, depressive episodes also has a family history of bipolar disorder, it would be in conflict with perhaps the most important scientific basis for the bipolar/unipolar distinction. Indeed, depressed patients with a family history of bipolar disorder, who have not experienced spontaneous manic or hypomanic episodes, are at increased risk of antidepressant-induced mania. Often, the apparent lack of spontaneous bipolar illness is simply a reflection of the patient's age: children or young adults suffering from what seems to be unipolar depression but who have a family history of bipolar disorder have a very high risk (more than 50%) of spontaneously developing manic episodes by age 30 (Geller et al. 2001; Goldberg et al. 2001). Thus, one should give a great deal of diagnostic weight to a family history of bipolar disorder.

Since bipolar disorder remains frequently misdiagnosed, and likely was more so in preceding generations (i.e., false-negative family histories), some attention should be paid to family histories of severe depression, substance abuse, suicide, past hospitalizations for mental illness, and electroconvulsive therapy (ECT). Such histories suggest severe mental illness, with bipolar disorder being a common condition that may have presented in those ways in the past.

Treatment Nonresponse

Further detail regarding treatment response will be found in Chapter 7, "Antidepressants in Bipolar Depression." In that chapter, evidence is provided to support the associations listed in Table 1–3. Here, we need

TABLE 1–3.   Differences in antidepressant treatment response between bipolar and unipolar depression

More common in bipolar than in unipolar depression:
  Antidepressant-induced mania
  Antidepressant-induced psychosis, mixed states, or suicidality
  Acute nonresponse
  Tolerance
  Rapid cycling

only note that antidepressant-induced mania is substantially more common in bipolar than in unipolar depression, occurring in about 20%–50% of persons with bipolar disorder versus in less than 1% of persons with unipolar depression (Akiskal et al. 2003; Ghaemi et al. 2004b).

An interesting clinical question is whether there are variations to antidepressant-induced mania that may not meet classic mania definitions. For instance, antidepressants could induce subthreshold, hypomanic states, often characterized primarily by irritability (Goldberg and Truman 2003), which could then become chronic (El-Mallakh and Karippot 2005). Antidepressants could also potentially lead to subsyndromal depressive or manic states (what has been termed *roughening*; Sachs 1996).

Manic symptoms induced by antidepressants are often mixed states. Since mixed states are associated with suicidality, the possibility exists that many cases of antidepressant-induced suicidality in children and adults (Khan et al. 2000; Murray et al. 2005; van Praag 2002) may represent the induction of mixed states in persons with undetected bipolar illness or a variant of bipolar illness.

New research also suggests that patients with bipolar disorder may be less likely to respond to antidepressants for the acute major depressive episode than those with unipolar depression (Ghaemi et al. 2004b), though other data conflict (Moller and Grunze 2000).

One study has examined the frequency of tolerance (initial response followed by later relapse into depression despite maintenance of antidepressant treatment) and found much higher rates of tolerance in bipolar than in unipolar depression (58% vs. 18%, respectively) (Ghaemi et al. 2004b). Lastly, a growing but still somewhat controversial literature (reviewed in Ghaemi et al. 2003) suggests that antidepressants may induce rapid cycling and cause increased mood episodes over time in bipolar illness, but not in unipolar depression (Ghaemi et al. 2004b).

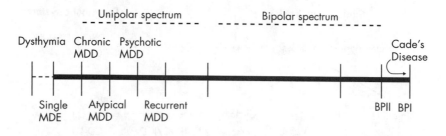

FIGURE 1–1. The manic–depressive spectrum.

Note. Cade's Disease is a term Terrence Ketter, M.D., first suggested to identify classical bipolar disorder, type I (discovered in 1949 by John Cade), which is often highly responsive to lithium (personal communication, July 2001). Abbreviations: BPI=bipolar disorder type I, BPII=bipolar disorder type II, MDD=major depressive disorder, MDE=major depressive episode.

Source. Reprinted from Ghaemi SN, Ko JY, Goodwin FK: "Cade's Disease and Beyond: Misdiagnosis, Antidepressant Use, and a Proposed Definition for Bipolar Spectrum Disorder." *Canadian Journal of Psychiatry,* 47:125–134, 2002. Used with permission.

THE BIPOLAR SPECTRUM

The above discussion of ways to differentiate bipolar from unipolar depression is also relevant to the general concept of a bipolar spectrum. The notion of a bipolar spectrum begins from the fact that many patients do not meet classical definitions of unipolar depression or bipolar disorder type I or II. As shown in Figure 1–1, many patients appear to demonstrate features of bipolarity such as the depressive phenomenology or the illness course mentioned above, and yet the inability to diagnose spontaneous manic or hypomanic episodes precludes the diagnosis of bipolar disorder types I or II.

It is important to realize that the bipolar spectrum concept, though relatively new (as resuscitated in recent years primarily by Akiskal; Akiskal 1996), is derived from Kraepelin's original manic-depressive illness concept (see Figure 1–2) (Kraepelin 1921). In Kraepelin's view, the key feature of manic-depressive illness—both the bipolar and recurrent unipolar forms—was recurrence. This contrasts with the current nosology (since DSM-III in 1980), which views polarity as the primary basis for diagnosing these mood disorders. In other words, the number of mood episodes the patient experienced, not what type of mood episode, was what mattered to Kraepelin. For DSM-III onward, what matters is the polarity of the episode (manic or depressive) and little else.

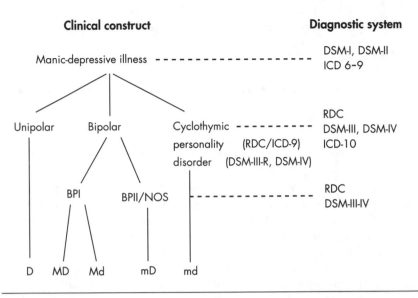

FIGURE 1–2. The evolution of the bipolar/unipolar distinction from manic–depressive illness.

Note. BPI=bipolar disorder type I, BPII= bipolar disorder type II, D=major depression, d=subsyndromal depression, M=mania, m=hypomania, NOS=not otherwise specified, RDC=Research Diagnostic Criteria.

Source. Reprinted from Goodwin FK, Ghaemi SN: "An introduction and history of affective disorders," in *Oxford Textbook of Psychiatry,* Vol 1. Gelder MG, Lopez-Ibor JJ Jr, Andreasen NC. Oxford, England, Oxford University Press, 2000, pp 677–680. Used with permission.

Various methods of classifying this bipolar spectrum have been proposed. One approach has been to provide further subtypes of bipolar illness (types III, IV, and so on) (Akiskal 2002). We have suggested another approach, which would be to combine all the further bipolar spectrum subtypes into a general category called "bipolar spectrum disorder"(BSD) (Ghaemi et al. 2002). A heuristic definition of BSD is provided in Table 1–4. Early research suggests that it may be a useful diagnosis that captures many patients with depressive disorders who are currently simply labeled as unipolar depressed patients. In one study of 87 consecutively referred young adults in an outpatient clinic, 83.9% were diagnosed with unipolar depression according to DSM-IV-TR. When bipolar spectrum disorder criteria were used, 47.1% of the total cohort were diagnosable with BSD (Smith et al. 2005). In one study of 61 patients with treatment refractory unipolar depression, 52% of the DSM-IV-TR unipolar group were diagnosable under this definition of BSD (Sharma et al. 2005).

TABLE 1–4.   A proposed definition of bipolar spectrum disorder

A. At least one major depressive episode
B. No spontaneous hypomanic or manic episodes
C. Either of the following, plus at least two items from criterion D, or both of the following plus one item from criterion D:
   1. A family history of bipolar disorder in a first degree relative
   2. Antidepressant-induced mania or hypomania
D. If no items from criterion C are present, six of the following nine criteria are needed:
   1. Hyperthymic personality (at baseline, nondepressed state)
   2. Recurrent major depressive episodes (>3)
   3. Brief major depressive episodes (on average, <3 months)
   4. Atypical depressive symptoms (DSM-IV-TR criteria)
   5. Psychotic major depressive episodes
   6. Early age at onset of major depressive episode (<age 25)
   7. Postpartum depression
   8. Antidepressant wear-off (acute but not prophylactic response)
   9. Lack of response to ≥3 antidepressant treatment trials

Source.   Reprinted from Ghaemi SN, Ko JY, Goodwin FK: "The Bipolar Spectrum and the Antidepressant View of the World." *Journal of Psychiatric Practice* 7:287–297, 2001. Used with permission.

Future clinical research will need to clarify whether it makes sense to keep a very broad and heterogeneous definition of unipolar depression in contrast with a very narrow and homogeneous definition of bipolar disorder. These studies suggest that some further broadening of the bipolar concept makes scientific and clinical sense.

DIAGNOSTIC CONTROVERSIES

Misdiagnosis

Numerous clinical studies now confirm that about 40% of persons with bipolar disorder are initially misdiagnosed with unipolar depression (Ghaemi et al. 2001). In some cases, the problem is not so much misdiagnosis as it is the natural history of the illness: if depressive episodes precede manic episodes, then the current nosology, correctly applied, would lead to misdiagnosis. This is sometimes called *pseudounipolar depression*. However, about 90% of patients with bipolar disorder will have a manic episode by the time they experience three major depressive episodes (Goodwin and Jamison 1990), so at some point clinicians would have the opportunity to observe and diagnose manic episodes.

Further, at least one clinical study corrects for the pseudounipolar natural history problem and finds a 37% misdiagnosis rate (Ghaemi et al. 2000).

Besides the clinical studies mentioned above, surveys of patients with bipolar disorder support a 50% or higher rate of misdiagnosis (Hirschfeld et al. 2003b; Lish et al. 1994). Both a survey and clinical studies indicate that it takes about a decade from the time patients seek help from mental health professionals for bipolar illness to be correctly diagnosed (shorter for type I illness; longer for type II) (Ghaemi et al. 2000).

Another reason leading to misdiagnosis may be that many patients prefer to see psychologists or social workers before they agree to see psychiatrists. In the only study to compare the groups, twice as many non-M.D. mental health professionals were seen as M.D.s (namely, psychiatrists) before the bipolar diagnosis was made (Ghaemi et al. 2000). That study revealed that it took non-M.D. mental health professionals an average of 8.9 years to diagnose bipolar disorder, while the psychiatrists on average made the diagnosis in 6.5 years (a comparison of bad and worse).

Currently, many patients with depressive illness are treated by their primary care practitioners and the frequency of misdiagnosis in this setting is not known. Self-report scales (like the Mood Disorder Questionnaire [MDQ]) have been used to study this topic, though they are not necessarily accurate diagnostic measures in such settings and are better seen as limited proxies for clinical diagnosis. With those caveats, one such study suggests a 91% misdiagnosis rate of bipolar disorder in the primary care setting (Das et al. 2005). Another study reports that only 80.2% of 85,358 patients in the community who screened MDQ positive for possible bipolar disorder were actually diagnosed and treated for it (Hirschfeld et al. 2003a). This is interesting—although it can be assumed that some of those patients may have been mistakenly identified by the MDQ, it is highly unlikely that a vast majority of them were mistaken.

Therefore, it is reasonable to conclude that in clinical mental health settings, about one-half of persons with bipolar disorder will be initially misdiagnosed for about a decade. In primary care medical settings, the misdiagnosis rate is likely worse.

Finally, the diagnostic criteria themselves may predispose bipolar disorder to misdiagnosis. Amin et al. (1999) found that a diagnosis of bipolar disorder was maintained at a 3-year follow-up in 91% of patients diagnosed according to ICD-10 criteria but only 78% of those patients diagnosed according to DSM-IV criteria. These discrepancies may be due to the fact that the DSM-IV schema defines the episode more reli-

---

TABLE 1–5. Reasons for the misdiagnosis of bipolar disorder

- The polarity-based approach to nosology
- Lack of insight by patients into mania
- Lack of knowledge by clinicians regarding manic symptoms
- The prototype approach to clinical diagnosis
- Poor memory during acute depressive episodes
- Clinicians' avoidance of family members and other treaters

---

ably than the disorder. This method therefore excludes the important characteristics of the natural course, longitudinal patterns, or recurrent history of the illness.

In sum, the state of diagnosis of bipolar disorder is hardly commendable. It is somewhat disheartening to note that in the past decade, despite an increase in research, writing, discussion, and continuing education activities about bipolar disorder, the misdiagnosis rate has held steady, with no sign of improvement (Hirschfeld et al. 2003b).

Important reasons for misdiagnosis are outlined in Table 1–5. Perhaps the most important factor that leads to misdiagnosis of bipolar disorder is lack of insight: as described earlier, about one-half of acutely manic patients do not realize they are experiencing a manic episode. Hence when a patient presents with depression and the DSM-trained clinician seeks to identify past mania or hypomania, the patient will deny such symptoms half of the time.

Consequently, the structure of DSM-IV-TR makes the misdiagnosis of bipolar disorder likely because of the requirement that mania be identified, even though patients frequently lack the understanding that they've been manic in the past. As seen in Figure 1–3, patients present in depression, and clinicians may either not obtain an accurate history of mania, or, frequently, they simply do not ask about manic symptoms. This leads to the diagnosis of unipolar depression. Instead, secondary and bipolar depression needs to be ruled out *before* unipolar depression is diagnosed. In the depressed patient, unipolar depression should be a diagnosis of exclusion—the last diagnosis made, not the first.

Overdiagnosis

Despite the evidence that bipolar misdiagnosis has not decreased in the past decade, some clinicians and researchers express concern about possible overdiagnosis of bipolar disorder. This concern is especially voiced in relation to discussion of broadening the definition of the bipolar spectrum.

Differential diagnosis of depression

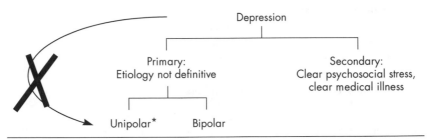

FIGURE 1–3. How the polarity-based approach to bipolar disorder in DSM-IV-TR can lead to misdiagnosis.

*A diagnosis of exclusion.

Source. From Goodwin FK, Ghaemi SN: "An Introduction and History of Affective Disorders," in *Oxford Textbook of Psychiatry,* Vol 1. Edited by Gelder MG, Lopez-Ibor JJ Jr, Andreasen NC. Oxford, England, Oxford University Press, 2000, pp 677–680.

In contrast to the extensive literature described above that supports the notion of continued underdiagnosis of bipolar disorder, there is a much more limited body of literature providing empirical evidence of overdiagnosis of bipolar disorder. A MEDLINE search of "overdiagnosis" and "misdiagnosis" for bipolar disorder identifies only three reports of possible overdiagnoses of bipolar disorder, two of which are case reports in letters to the editor. In the only published study (Krasa and Tolbert 1994), of 53 adolescents admitted with a clinical diagnosis of bipolar disorder, 72% met DSM-III-R criteria, suggesting that 28% were mistakenly diagnosed with the condition. As noted below, however, it is controversial whether DSM criteria for bipolar disorder, developed through study of adults, are equally applicable in pediatric populations. In the cases reported as possible overdiagnoses, one is not easily convinced that those patients indeed do not have bipolar disorder. For instance, it appears that the main reason why the author of one letter to the editor thought that the patient did not have bipolar disorder is due to lack of response to divalproex and a good response to antidepressants (Hutto 2001). Of course, medication response is quite nonspecific and, though informative, is not useful as the sole source of data for diagnostic validity.

As noted throughout this chapter, multiple sources of data are needed to establish diagnostic validity. Other studies, albeit with a broader approach to bipolar diagnosis than in DSM-IV-TR (i.e., excluding the duration requirements), report much higher rates of underdiagnosis of bipolar disorder in children. In one study of 82 children (mean age 10.6 years) diagnosed with DSM-IV-TR criteria but excluding the duration requirements, 90% had not been previously diagnosed with bipolar disorder (Faedda et al. 2004a).

In searching for possible unpublished data regarding the diagnosis of bipolar disorder, we identified a poster presented at a bipolar conference in which 70 adult inpatients with clinical diagnoses of bipolar disorder were rediagnosed using a structured clinical interview for DSM-IV-TR (SCID) in preparation for a research study (Berns et al. 2003). Only 78% were diagnosed, on the basis of DSM-IV-TR criteria, with any form of bipolar disorder. Interestingly, the researchers also observed that some patients hospitalized with nonbipolar diagnoses appeared likely to have bipolar disorder. In seven cases where such underdiagnosis was suspected, five indeed met bipolar disorder criteria with a SCID interview. Hence the authors found evidence of both overdiagnosis and underdiagnosis. The latter study partly confirms the earlier study in adolescence, suggesting that some patients are mistakenly diagnosed with bipolar disorder. If these estimates are correct, we might conclude that about 25% of hospitalized patients diagnosed with bipolar disorder may not have the condition, according to current DSM-IV-TR criteria. On the other hand, about 40% of patients with bipolar disorder, when DSM-IV-TR criteria are used, are initially misdiagnosed with other conditions. Thus underdiagnosis still seems to be more of a problem than overdiagnosis.

Of course, besides the issue of under- or overdiagnosis using our current criteria, there is the larger issue of whether current DSM-IV-TR criteria for bipolar disorder are valid. This is the problem of the bipolar spectrum whose solution will require better clinical and epidemiological research, along with better nosologically oriented genetic and neurobiological research.

Children and Adolescents

The question of diagnosis of bipolar depression in children is both quite complex and quite simple. To start with the simple aspect of the problem, bipolar disorder, as noted above, has an earlier age at onset than unipolar depression. As previously described, data from a study of children with mean age of 12.3 experiencing depression suggests that about one-half develop bipolar disorder by age 21 (Geller et al. 2001). Thus, the question of bipolar disorder in children is simply the question of depression: if children are depressed, the likelihood of bipolar disorder is high, perhaps about 50%. If a depressed child also has a family history of bipolar disorder, then the likelihood of bipolar disorder is even higher.

Therefore, in depressed children, clinicians should have a high index of suspicion that the illness is bipolar disorder, even if manic or hypomanic episodes have not been demonstrated yet.

The complex part of the problem is whether DSM-IV-TR criteria for mania, developed in adults, are applicable to children. At one level, it would seem logical that adult criteria do not apply in the same way to children. In order to establish the childhood criteria for bipolar disorder, research in children is required, with follow-up into adulthood. Such research has begun, and the developing evidence seems to fall into two categories: In one line of findings, it has been suggested that bipolar disorder in children is best established with the presence of elation, grandiosity, decreased need for sleep, racing thoughts, and hypersexuality (Geller et al. 2002). While most clinicians would agree with that definition, the more controversial question is whether other children might have manic presentations without elation and grandiosity, but rather primarily with irritability of mood and aggressive behavior (Wozniak et al. 1995). Clinical experience, dating back to Kraepelin (Trede et al. 2005), and recent research with adults (Cassidy and Carroll 2001) suggest that irritability and aggressive behavior are indeed important components of manic episodes in many patients; furthermore, it appears that euphoric mania represents a minority of manic episodes in adults, with mixed and irritable moods predominating (Cassidy and Carroll 2001). In fact, children may be especially sensitive to developing serotonin reuptake inhibitor (SRI)–induced mania, perhaps more so than adults (Baldessarini et al. 2005). Hence, it would not be surprising if manic episodes in children might also present primarily with irritability rather than euphoria. However, unless a few other manic criteria are present, the DSM-IV-TR definition would not be currently met, leading to the current controversy. Follow-up of such children into adulthood will provide the best evidence of whether such presentations in children indeed represent a childhood variation on bipolar disorder.

Attention-Deficit/Hyperactivity Disorder in Children and Adults

In children, a major diagnostic issue is differentiating attention-deficit/ hyperactivity disorder (ADHD) and bipolar disorder, which is a challenge largely because of the overlapping symptoms of distractibility and hyperactivity. In one study, about 90% of children who met DSM-III-R criteria for bipolar disorder also met criteria for ADHD. In contrast, only about 25% of those who presented with ADHD met criteria for bipolar disorder (Wozniak et al. 1995). Thus, it appears that many children are diagnosable with ADHD alone and seem to respond well to stimulants, while some children who appear to have ADHD may in fact have bipolar disorder. This observation is supported by research indicating that about 9.5% of adults with bipolar disorder can be retrospectively diagnosable with ADHD in childhood (Nierenberg et al. 2005). The use of stimulants, while not diagnostic, can be informative in the setting of other possible manic symptoms and a family history of bipolar disorder. In such children, stimulants are frequently ineffective, are limited in efficacy, or can trigger manic episodes associated with marked irritability and aggression. In one study of 82 children (mean age 10.6 years), 18% appeared to develop mania with amphetamines, though the rate of mania with other antidepressants was higher (44%) (Faedda et al. 2004b). One study found that children with bipolar disorder who were treated with stimulants had an earlier age at onset to their bipolar illness than children with bipolar disorder who had never received stimulants (DelBello et al. 2001). Although this outcome might have been influenced by other factors, one possibility is that stimulants speed the onset of bipolar illness, essentially worsening the course of the illness. Neurodevelopmental risks of stimulant use in long-term treatment of young animals have also been reported (Bolanos et al. 2003) and need to be weighed against the limited benefits in children with risk factors for bipolar disorder (Volkow and Insel 2003).

Therefore, we would generally recommend caution in the diagnosis of ADHD in children and especially in the use of stimulants for treatment of this disorder. In the first nationwide, community-based survey of ADHD diagnoses in the United States (Centers for Disease Control and Prevention 2005), it was found that 7.8% of children ages 4–17 were diagnosed with ADHD in 2003. ADHD was diagnosed in males much more often than in females (11.0% vs. 4.4%), and diagnosed in children ages 9–17 twice as often as in children ages 4–8 (9.7% vs. 4.1%). Children were also more likely to receive the diagnosis if they were white, insured, and below the federal poverty level. About half of those who received the diagnosis of ADHD were given stimulants (4.3%); again, even more so males than females (6.2% vs. 2.4%). The evidence for overdiagnosis of ADHD presented in other studies is somewhat supported by the finding of notable regional differences in diagnoses. The diagnosis of ADHD was more likely in states with the highest poverty levels (highest diagnosis rates of 10%–11% were in Alabama, Louisiana, and West Virginia) compared to wealthier states (lowest diagnosis rates of 5%–5.5% were in Colorado and California). Since there is obviously no biological reason why living in Alabama should predispose one to ADHD more than living in Colorado, social and economic factors leading to diagnosis and treatment appear relevant.

Despite the limitations in diagnosing and treating ADHD in children, the evidence for the validity of the diagnosis and the utility of treatment, in those appropriately diagnosed, is much more extensive than in adults. Yet the diagnosis of adult ADHD has become quite popular, coinciding with the marketing of the first medication for adult ADHD, Strattera (atomoxitene), by the pharmaceutical industry in 2002. Although there is some research on the potential validity of adult ADHD, that research is much more limited than childhood ADHD and awaits replication by independent research groups.

In the past, it was generally considered that ADHD did not persist into adulthood. Despite the recent surge of interest in adult ADHD, a recent review supporting the notion of adult ADHD only cited two studies (Wilens et al. 2004). One was a 1985 study of 63 children followed for 15 years that reported that a minority of the children continued to have symptoms into young adulthood (Weiss et al. 1985). Another study involved a 6-year follow-up of adolescents and reported improvement in hyperactivity but some persistence of attentional deficits (Achenbach et al. 1998). Compared with the century-old extensive literature on bipolar disorder (Trede et al. 2005), these data on the course of illness that support the validity of the concept of adult ADHD appear far from convincing, suggesting even more caution in diagnosing and treating adult ADHD.

It is worth noting that adult patients often seeking amphetamine stimulants for ADHD may be engaging in substance abuse. In addition to obtaining an adequate history of past substance use, clinicians may need to discuss with all patients the fact that improvement in attention in response to amphetamine stimulant treatment does not validate a diagnosis of ADHD. As noted earlier, treatment response is one of only four diagnostic validators, and it is the weakest and most nonspecific of them. This is especially the case when one is faced with a drug of abuse. The reason that amphetamines are abused is because they improve attention in normal people, irrespective of any diagnosis (Miller et al. 1989). Thus, such improvement is not diagnostically relevant.

Personality Disorders

Another topic of heated controversy is whether bipolar disorder is overdiagnosed at the expense of personality disorders, such as borderline personality disorder (Akiskal 2004; Birnbaum 2004; Magill 2004; Paris 2004; Smith et al. 2004). While this argument has been made based on case reports (Bolton and Gunderson 1996), no empirical evidence has been published to that effect. On the other hand, there is extensive research that borderline personality disorder is overdiagnosed in patients with abnormal and/or unstable moods, with frequent resolution of "borderline" traits when the mood episode resolves with antidepressants or mood stabilizers (Frankenburg and Zanarini 2002; Preston et al. 2004). Thus, the empirical evidence again seems to suggest a need to abstain from diagnosing borderline personality disorder in individuals with major depressive and manic or hypomanic episodes. Instead, it makes sense clinically to treat their mood episodes. If those episodes resolve and the individual continues to have borderline personality disorder traits in the euthymic state, then a true comorbidity may exist.

On the other hand, there certainly are individuals without hypomanic or manic episodes but who have long-standing and unchanging borderline personality traits. Those persons are best diagnosed and treated primarily with psychotherapies for borderline personality disorder. Mood lability in that setting, not meeting hypomania or mania syndromal definitions, is often a feature of the borderline personality condition. Although some data suggest that mood lability in general may be a predictor of bipolar disorder (Benazzi and Akiskal 2005a), it seems reasonable to emphasize the classic approach of requiring other symptoms to meet syndromal definitions of mood episodes (whether in the narrow DSM-IV-TR model or the broader bipolar spectrum disorder model).

Our perspective is that we need to recognize overlap of the two syndromes where such overlap exists, while also working hard diagnostically to identify those who predominantly have bipolar disorder in some cases or predominantly borderline personality disorder in other cases. This approach is supported by some of the limited, empirical evidence on the borderline/bipolar issue. In patients with bipolar disorder type II, Benazzi found that there was extensive overlap of borderline traits of affective instability, but not with borderline criteria for impulsivity (Benazzi 2005). Similar results were found in a previous study by another group (Henry et al. 2001a). Thus, mood lability is not a useful diagnostic feature to distinguish the two conditions, but borderline-type impulsive behaviors (such as cutting) are much less common in bipolar disorder. When clinicians simply pay attention to standard definitions of mania and hypomania, most patients with bipolar disorder, even type II, can reasonably be distinguished from borderline personality disorder (Benazzi 2000).

Again the key is to get beyond simply symptom overlap, such as mood lability, and use the other diagnostic validators, especially course and family history, as described throughout this chapter (Paris 2004).

Mixed States and Suicide

The association of potential, increased risk of suicide in some persons treated with antidepressants raises the question of whether those depressed patients might have instead experienced mixed states. If a broader definition of mixed states, as described earlier, is valid, then many individuals today diagnosed with major depressive episodes instead might be experiencing depressive mixed states. Antidepressants can cause mixed episodes (Dilsaver and Swann 1995) or worsen them, and the limited data available indicate that antidepressants do not improve depressive symptoms in mixed episodes (Prien et al. 1984). Mixed episodes are known to be associated with a high degree of suicidality, perhaps even more so than anergic pure depression (Dilsaver et al. 1994).

Thus, it is not unlikely that many of the depressed children who entered clinical trials with SRI antidepressants actually had bipolar disorder, given the data that about half will likely develop manic or hypomanic episodes (Geller et al. 2001). They would then likely be predisposed to antidepressant-induced mixed episodes, with concomitant suicidality (Berk and Dodd 2005). As discussed previously, similar risks would likely hold for young adults in their 20s (Goldberg et al. 2001).

A related issue is the fact that many clinicians appear to misdiagnose mixed episodes as pure depressive episodes, and then provide treatment with antidepressants. Data supporting the use of antidepressants for depressive mixed episodes are very limited (Brown et al. 1994; Rihmer et al. 1998), but this has not seemed to deter clinicians from this practice. On the other hand, anticonvulsants and antipsychotic agents are likely much more effective (Bowden et al. 1994; Sachs et al. 2002) and need to be more seriously considered for depressive mixed states to the extent that they can be shown to be distinct from pure major depression. In sum, it could be that the problem of antidepressant-induced suicidality may really be the tip of an iceberg of inappropriately treated bipolar depression and depressive mixed states.

SUMMARY

Bipolar depression is the "other" depression that is quite common and often confused with unipolar depression. There are important nosological differences between the presentations of bipolar and unipolar depression, and the misdiagnosis of bipolar depression as unipolar is a major clinical problem that needs attention. In this chapter, we focused on those differences—particularly in depressive phenomenology, course, family history, and antidepressant nonresponse. The concept of the bipolar spectrum also is important heuristically and may be validated by further nosological research. Several important diagnostic controversies will need elucidation by further research.

REFERENCES

Achenbach TM, Howell CT, McConaughy SH, et al: Six-year predictors of problems in a national sample: IV. Young adult signs of disturbance. J Am Acad Child Adolesc Psychiatry 37:718–727, 1998

Agosti V, Stewart JW: Atypical and non-atypical subtypes of depression: comparison of social functioning, symptoms, course of illness, co-morbidity, and demographic features. J Affect Disord 65:75–79, 2001

Akiskal HS: The prevalent clinical spectrum of bipolar disorders: beyond DSM-IV. J Clin Psychopharmacol 16 (suppl 1):4S–14S, 1996

Akiskal HS: Classification, diagnosis and boundaries of bipolar disorders, in Bipolar Disorder. Edited by Maj M, Akiskal H, Lopez-Ibor J, et al. London, Wiley, 2002, pp 1–52

Akiskal HS: Demystifying borderline personality: critique of the concept and unorthodox reflections on its natural kinship with the bipolar spectrum. Acta Psychiatr Scand 110:401–407, 2004

Akiskal HS, Benazzi F, Perugi G, et al: Agitated "unipolar" depression reconceptualized as a depressive mixed state: implications for the antidepressant-suicide controversy. J Affect Disord 85:245–258, 2005

Akiskal HS, Bourgeois ML, Angst J, et al: Re-evaluating the prevalence of and diagnostic composition within the broad clinical spectrum of bipolar disorders. J Affect Disord 59 (suppl 1):S5–S30, 2000

Akiskal HS, Hantouche EG, Allilaire JF, et al: Validating antidepressant-associated hypomania (bipolar III): a systematic comparison with spontaneous hypomania (bipolar II). J Affect Disord 73:65–74, 2003

Akiskal HS, Maser JD, Zeller PJ, et al: Switching from "unipolar" to bipolar II. An 11-year prospective study of clinical and temperamental predictors in 559 patients. Arch Gen Psychiatry 52:114–123, 1995

Amin S, Singh SP, Brewin J, et al: Diagnostic stability of first-episode psychosis. Comparison of ICD-10 and DSM-III-R systems. Br J Psychiatry 175:537–543, 1999

Baldessarini RJ, Faedda GL, Hennen J: Risk of mania with antidepressants. Arch Pediatr Adolesc Med 159:298, 2005

Benazzi F: Prevalence and clinical features of atypical depression in depressed outpatients: a 467-case study. Psychiatry Res 86:259–265, 1999

Benazzi F: Borderline personality disorder and bipolar II disorder in private practice depressed outpatients. Compr Psychiatry 41:106–110, 2000

Benazzi F: The clinical picture of bipolar II outpatient depression in private practice. Psychopathology 34:81–84, 2001a

Benazzi F: Depressive mixed state: testing different definitions. Psychiatry Clin Neurosci 55:647–652, 2001b

Benazzi F: Depressive mixed state: a feature of the natural course of bipolar II (and major depressive) disorder? Psychopathology 37:207–212, 2004a

Benazzi F: Is depressive mixed state a transition between depression and hypomania? Eur Arch Psychiatry Clin Neurosci 254:69–75, 2004b

Benazzi F: Borderline personality–bipolar spectrum relationship. Prog Neuropsychopharmacol Biol Psychiatry, 2005

Benazzi F, Akiskal HS: A downscaled practical measure of mood lability as a screening tool for bipolar II. J Affect Disord 84:225–232, 2005a

Benazzi F, Akiskal HS: Irritable-hostile depression: further validation as a bipolar depressive mixed state. J Affect Disord 84:197–207, 2005b

Benazzi F, Koukopoulos A, Akiskal HS: Toward a validation of a new definition of agitated depression as a bipolar mixed state (mixed depression). Eur Psychiatry 19:85–90, 2004

Berk M, Dodd S: Are treatment emergent suicidality and decreased response to antidepressants in younger patients due to bipolar disorder being misdiagnosed as unipolar depression? Med Hypotheses 65:39–43, 2005

Berns S, Jaeger J, Iannuzzo R, et al: A comparison of medical chart diagnosis with SCID consensus diagnosis among bipolar disorder patients (abstract), in Fifth International Conference on Bipolar Disorder. Edited by Soares JC, Gershon S. Pittsburgh, PA, Blackwell Munksgaard, 2003, p 33

Birnbaum RJ: Borderline, bipolar, or both? Harv Rev Psychiatry 12:146–149, 2004

Bolanos CA, Barrot M, Berton O, et al. Methylphenidate treatment during pre- and periadolescence alters behavioral responses to emotional stimuli at adulthood. Biol Psychiatry 54:1317–1329, 2003

Bolton S, Gunderson JG: Distinguishing borderline personality disorder from bipolar disorder: differential diagnosis and implications. Am J Psychiatry 153:1202–1207, 1996

Bowden C, Brugger A, Swann A, et al: Efficacy of divalproex vs lithium and placebo in the treatment of mania. JAMA 271:918–924, 1994

Boylan KR, Bieling PJ, Marriott M, et al: Impact of comorbid anxiety disorders on outcome in a cohort of patients with bipolar disorder. J Clin Psychiatry 65:1106–1113, 2004

Brown ES, Dilsaver SC, Shoaib AM, et al: Depressive mania: response of residual depression to bupropion. Biol Psychiatry 35:493–494, 1994

Cantor N, Smith EE, French RS, et al: Psychiatric diagnosis as prototype categorization. J Abnorm Psychol 89:181–193, 1980

Cassano GB, Akiskal HS, Savino M, et al: Proposed subtypes of bipolar II and related disorders: with hypomanic episodes (or cyclothymia) and with hyperthymic temperament. J Affect Disord 26:127–140, 1992

Cassidy F, Carroll BJ: Frequencies of signs and symptoms in mixed and pure episodes of mania: implications for the study of manic episodes. Prog Neuropsychopharmacol Biol Psychiatry 25:659–665, 2001

Centers for Disease Control and Prevention: Prevalence of diagnosis and medication treatment for attention-deficit/hyperactivity disorder—United States, 2003. MMWR Morb Mortal Wkly Rep 54:842–847, 2005

Chiaroni P, Hantouche EG, Gouvernet J, et al: Hyperthymic and depressive temperaments study in controls, as a function of their familial loading for mood disorders. Encephale 30:509–515, 2004

Das AK, Olfson M, Gameroff MJ, et al: Screening for bipolar disorder in a primary care practice. JAMA 293:956–963, 2005

DelBello MP, Soutullo CA, Hendricks W, et al: Prior stimulant treatment in adolescents with bipolar disorder: association with age at onset. Bipolar Disord 3:53–57, 2001

Dell'Osso L, Pini S, Cassano GB, et al: Insight into illness in patients with mania, mixed mania, bipolar depression and major depression with psychotic features. Bipolar Disord 4:315–322, 2002

Dilsaver SC, Swann AC: Mixed mania: apparent induction by a tricyclic antidepressant in five consecutively treated patients with bipolar depression. Biol Psychiatry 37:60–62, 1995

Dilsaver S, Chen Y, Swann A, et al: Suicidality in patients with pure and depressive mania. Am J Psychiatry 151:1312–1315, 1994

Dube S, Andersen SW, Sofia P, et al: Meta-analysis of olanzapine-fluoxetine in treatment-resistant depression (abstract). Presented at the annual meeting of the American Psychiatric Association (May 8–13). Philadelphia, PA, 2002

El-Mallakh RS, Karippot A: Antidepressant-associated chronic irritable dysphoria (acid) in bipolar disorder: a case series. J Affect Disord 84:267–272, 2005

Faedda GL, Baldessarini RJ, Glovinsky IP, et al: Pediatric bipolar disorder: phenomenology and course of illness. Bipolar Disord 6:305–313, 2004a

Faedda GL, Baldessarini RJ, Glovinsky IP, et al: Treatment-emergent mania in pediatric bipolar disorder: a retrospective case review. J Affect Disord 82:149–158, 2004b

Frankenburg FR, Zanarini MC: Divalproex sodium treatment of women with borderline personality disorder and bipolar II disorder: a double-blind placebo-controlled pilot study. J Clin Psychiatry 63:442–446, 2002

Freeman MP, Keck PE Jr, McElroy SL: Postpartum depression with bipolar disorder. Am J Psychiatry 158:52, 2001

Geller B, Zimerman B, Williams M, et al: Bipolar disorder at prospective follow-up of adults who had prepubertal major depressive disorder. Am J Psychiatry 158:125–127, 2001

Geller B, Zimerman B, Williams M, et al: Phenomenology of prepubertal and early adolescent bipolar disorder: examples of elated mood, grandiose behaviors, decreased need for sleep, racing thoughts and hypersexuality. J Child Adolesc Psychopharmacol 12:3–9, 2002

Ghaemi SN: The Concepts of Psychiatry. Baltimore, MD, Johns Hopkins University Press, 2003

Ghaemi SN, Rosenquist KJ: Is insight in mania state-dependent? A meta-analysis. J Nerv Ment Dis 192:771–775, 2004

Ghaemi SN, Stoll AL, Pope HG: Lack of insight in bipolar disorder: The acute manic episode. J Nerv Ment Dis 183:464–467, 1995

Ghaemi SN, Boiman EE, Goodwin FK: Diagnosing bipolar disorder and the effect of antidepressants: a naturalistic study. J Clin Psychiatry 61:804–808, 2000

Ghaemi SN, Ko JY, Goodwin FK: The bipolar spectrum and the antidepressant view of the world. J Psychiatr Pract 7:287–297, 2001

Ghaemi SN, Ko JY, Goodwin FK: "Cade's disease" and beyond: misdiagnosis, antidepressant use, and a proposed definition for bipolar spectrum disorder. Can J Psychiatry 47:125–134, 2002

Ghaemi SN, Hsu DJ, Soldani F, et al: Antidepressants in bipolar disorder: the case for caution. Bipolar Disord 5:421–433, 2003

Ghaemi SN, Hsu DJ, Ko JY, et al: Bipolar spectrum disorder: a pilot study. Psychopathology 37:222–226, 2004a

Ghaemi SN, Rosenquist KJ, Ko JY, et al: Antidepressant treatment in bipolar versus unipolar depression. Am J Psychiatry 161:163–165, 2004b

Goldberg JF, Truman CJ: Antidepressant-induced mania: an overview of current controversies. Bipolar Disord 5:407–420, 2003

Goldberg JF, Harrow M, Whiteside JE: Risk for bipolar illness in patients initially hospitalized for unipolar depression. Am J Psychiatry 158:1265–1270, 2001

Goodwin F, Jamison K: Manic Depressive Illness. New York, Oxford University Press, 1990

Henry C, Mitropoulou V, New AS, et al: Affective instability and impulsivity in borderline personality and bipolar II disorders: similarities and differences. J Psychiatr Res 35:307–312, 2001a

Henry C, Sorbara F, Lacoste J, et al: Antidepressant-induced mania in bipolar patients: identification of risk factors. J Clin Psychiatry 62:249–255, 2001b

Hirschfeld RM, Calabrese JR, Weissman MM, et al: Screening for bipolar disorder in the community. J Clin Psychiatry 64:53–59, 2003a

Hirschfeld RM, Lewis L, Vornik LA: Perceptions and impact of bipolar disorder: how far have we really come? Results of the National Depressive and Manic-Depressive Association 2000 survey of individuals with bipolar disorder. J Clin Psychiatry 64:161–174, 2003b

Hutto B: Potential overdiagnosis of bipolar disorder. Psychiatr Serv 52:687–688, 2001

Janzarik W: Jaspers, Kurt Schneider and the Heidelberg school of psychiatry. Hist Psychiatry 9:241–252, 1998

Judd LL, Akiskal HS, Maser JD, et al: A prospective 12-year study of subsyndromal and syndromal depressive symptoms in unipolar major depressive disorders. Arch Gen Psychiatry 55:694–700, 1998

Keitner GI, Solomon DA, Ryan CE, et al: Prodromal and residual symptoms in bipolar I disorder. Compr Psychiatry 37:362–367, 1996

Kessing LV, Andersen PK, Mortensen PB: Recurrence in affective disorder, I: case register study. Br J Psychiatry 172:23–28, 1998

Khan A, Warne HA, Brown WA: Symptom reduction and suicide risk in patients treated with placebo in antidepressant clinical trials: an analysis of the Food and Drug Administration database. Arch Gen Psychiatry 57:311–317, 2000

Koukopoulos A, Koukopoulos A: Agitated depression as a mixed state and the problem of melancholia. Psychiatr Clin North Am 22:547–564, 1999

Kraepelin E: Manic-Depressive Insanity and Paranoia. Translated by Barclay RM and edited by Robertson GM. Edinburgh, Scotland, Livingstone, 1921 [Reprinted New York, Arno Press, 1976]

Krasa NR, Tolbert HA: Adolescent bipolar disorder: a nine-year experience. J Affect Disord 30:175–184, 1994

Leucht S, McGrath J, Kissling W: Lithium for schizophrenia. Cochrane Database Syst Rev, CD003834, 2003

Lish J, Dime-Meenan S, Whybrow P, et al: The National Depressive and Manic-Depressive Association (DMDA) survey of bipolar members. J Affect Disord 31:281–294, 1994

Magill CA: The boundary between borderline personality disorder and bipolar disorder: current concepts and challenges. Can J Psychiatry 49:551–556, 2004

Miller NS, Millman RB, Gold MS: Amphetamines: pharmacology, abuse and addiction. Adv Alcohol Subst Abuse 8:53–69, 1989

Mitchell P, Parker G, Jamieson K, et al: Are there any differences between bipolar and unipolar melancholia? J Affect Disord 25:97–105, 1992

Mitchell PB, Wilhelm K, Parker G, et al: The clinical features of bipolar depression: a comparison with matched major depressive disorder patients. J Clin Psychiatry 62:212–216, 2001

Moller HJ, Grunze H: Have some guidelines for the treatment of acute bipolar depression gone too far in the restriction of antidepressants? Eur Arch Psychiatry Clin Neurosci 250:57–68, 2000

Murray ML, Wong IC, Thompson M: Do selective serotonin reuptake inhibitors cause suicide? Antidepressant prescribing to children and adolescents by GPs has fallen since CSM advice. BMJ 330:1151, 2005

Nierenberg AA, Miyahara S, Spencer T, et al: Clinical and diagnostic implications of lifetime attention-deficit/hyperactivity disorder comorbidity in adults with bipolar disorder: data from the first 1,000 STEP-BD participants. Biol Psychiatry 57:1467–1473, 2005

Paris J: Borderline or bipolar? Distinguishing borderline personality disorder from bipolar spectrum disorders. Harv Rev Psychiatry 12:140–145, 2004

Parker G, Roy K, Wilhelm K, et al: The nature of bipolar depression: implications for the definition of melancholia. J Affect Disord 59:217–224, 2000

Perlis RH, Fraguas R, Fava M, et al: The prevalence and clinical correlates of anger attacks during depressive episodes in bipolar disorder. J Affect Disord 79:291–295, 2004

Perlis RH, Fraguas R, Fava M, et al: Prevalence and clinical correlates of irritability in major depressive disorder: a preliminary report from the Sequenced Treatment Alternatives to Relieve Depression study. J Clin Psychiatry 66:159–166; quiz 147, 273–274, 2005

Perris C: A study of bipolar (manic-depressive) and unipolar recurrent depressive psychoses. Acta Psychiatr Scand Suppl 194:15–152, 1966

Perugi G, Akiskal HS: The soft bipolar spectrum redefined: focus on the cyclothymic, anxious-sensitive, impulse-dyscontrol, and binge-eating connection in bipolar II and related conditions. Psychiatr Clin North Am 25:713–737, 2002

Perugi G, Akiskal HS, Micheli C, et al: Clinical subtypes of bipolar mixed states: validating a broader European definition in 143 cases. J Affect Disord 43:169–180, 1997

Perugi G, Toni C, Akiskal HS: Anxious-bipolar comorbidity. Diagnostic and treatment challenges. Psychiatr Clin North Am 22:565–583, viii, 1999

Perugi G, Maremmani I, Toni C, et al: The contrasting influence of depressive and hyperthymic temperaments on psychometrically derived manic subtypes. Psychiatry Res 101:249–258, 2001

Preston GA, Marchant BK, Reimherr FW, et al: Borderline personality disorder in patients with bipolar disorder and response to lamotrigine. J Affect Disord 79:297–303, 2004

Prien RF, Kupfer DJ, Mansky PA, et al: Drug therapy in the prevention of recurrences in unipolar and bipolar affective disorders. Report of the NIMH Collaborative Study Group comparing lithium carbonate, imipramine, and a lithium carbonate-imipramine combination. Arch Gen Psychiatry 41:1096–1104, 1984

Rihmer Z, Kiss GH, Kecskes I, et al: SSRI supplementation of antimanic medication in dysphoric mania. Pharmacopsychiatry 31:30–31, 1998

Robins E, Guze SB: Establishment of diagnostic validity in psychiatric illness: its application to schizophrenia. Am J Psychiatry 126:983–987, 1970

Sachs GS: Bipolar mood disorder: practical strategies for acute and maintenance phase treatment. J Clin Psychopharmacol 16:32S–47S, 1996

Sachs GS, Grossman F, Ghaemi SN, et al: Combination of a mood stabilizer with risperidone or haloperidol for treatment of acute mania: a double-blind, placebo-controlled comparison of efficacy and safety. Am J Psychiatry 159:1146–1154, 2002

Sato T, Bottlender R, Schroter A, et al: Frequency of manic symptoms during a depressive episode and unipolar 'depressive mixed state' as bipolar spectrum. Acta Psychiatr Scand 107:268–274, 2003

Schatzberg AF, Rothschild AJ: Psychotic (delusional) major depression: should it be included as a distinct syndrome in DSM-IV? Am J Psychiatry 149:733–745, 1992

Sharma V, Khan M, Smith A: A closer look at treatment resistant depression: is it due to a bipolar diathesis? J Affect Disord 84:251–257, 2005

Smith DJ, Muir WJ, Blackwood DH: Is borderline personality disorder part of the bipolar spectrum? Harv Rev Psychiatry 12:133–139, 2004

Smith DJ, Harrison N, Muir W, et al: The high prevalence of bipolar spectrum disorders in young adults with recurrent depression: toward an innovative diagnostic framework. J Affect Disord 84:167–178, 2005

Sprock J: Classification of schizoaffective disorder. Compr Psychiatry 29:55–71, 1988

Stephens JH, McHugh PR: Characteristics and long-term follow-up of patients hospitalized for mood disorders in the Phipps Clinic, 1913–1940. J Nerv Ment Disord 179:64–73, 1991

Tohen M, Waternaux CM, Tsuang M: Outcome in mania: a 4-year prospective follow-up of 75 patients utilizing survival analysis. Arch Gen Psychiatry 47:1106–1111, 1990

Tohen M, Vieta E, Calabrese J, et al: Efficacy of olanzapine and olanzapine-fluoxetine combination in the treatment of bipolar I depression. Arch Gen Psychiatry 60:1079–1088, 2003

Trede K, Salvatore P, Baethge C, et al: Manic-depressive illness: evolution in Kraepelin's Textbook, 1883–1926. Harv Rev Psychiatry 13:155–178, 2005

van Praag HM: Why has the antidepressant era not shown a significant drop in suicide rates? Crisis 23:77–82, 2002

Volkow ND, Insel TR: What are the long-term effects of methylphenidate treatment? Biol Psychiatry 54:1307–1309, 2003

Weiss G, Hechtman L, Milroy T: Psychiatric status of hyperactives as adults: a controlled prospective 15-year follow-up of 63 hyperactive children. J Am Acad Child Psychiatry 24:211–220, 1985

Westen D, Shedler J: A prototype matching approach to diagnosing personality disorders: toward DSM-V. J Personal Disord 14:109–126, 2000

Wilens TE, Faraone SV, Biederman J: Attention-deficit/hyperactivity disorder in adults. JAMA 292:619–623, 2004

Wolpert EA, Goldberg JF, Harrow M: Rapid cycling in unipolar and bipolar affective disorders. Am J Psychiatry 147:725–728, 1990

Wozniak J, Biederman J, Kiely K, et al: Mania-like symptoms suggestive of childhood-onset bipolar disorder in clinically referred children. J Am Acad Child Adolesc Psychiatry 34:867–876, 1995

BIOLOGY OF
BIPOLAR DEPRESSION

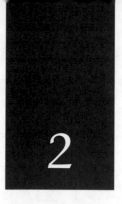

2

NEUROBIOLOGY OF BIPOLAR DEPRESSION

Alan C. Swann, M.D.

SPECIFICITY OF BIPOLAR DEPRESSION

The biology of bipolar depression encompasses depressive episodes of bipolar disorder and the biology of the underlying illness that gives rise to the depressive episodes. Understanding the biology of bipolar depression should increase the effectiveness of its diagnosis and treatment. In our current nosology, mania or hypomania is required for diagnosis of bipolar disorder (First et al. 1996). Yet, for most patients, depression is the most salient feature of the illness: the average patient with bipolar disorder spends three times as much time depressed as manic (Post et al. 2003), and depressive episodes are associated with most of the psychosocial impairment of bipolar disorder and with mortality from suicide (MacQueen et al. 2000). Bipolar disorder usually starts with depression, rather than with mania or hypomania, often resulting in a substantial period of misdiagnosed illness and a course of illness that is worse than when mania is the first episode (Perugi et al. 2000). Therefore, it should be our goal to identify bipolar disorder before the first manic episode.

Figure 2–1 shows four possible models for specificity of bipolar depression: 1) bipolar and unipolar depressions could be distinct clinical and biological syndromes, 2) biologically distinct bipolar and unipolar depressions could appear clinically similar in the two illnesses, 3) depression could be a nonspecific, biological and clinical syndrome super-

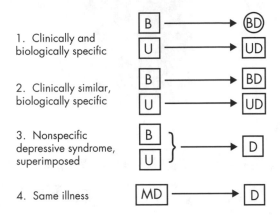

FIGURE 2–1.   Models for bipolar depression specificity.

Note.   Four models for specificity of relationships between depressive episodes and bipolar disorder. Abbreviations: B=bipolar, D=depression, M=mania, U=unipolar.

imposed on either bipolar or unipolar disorder, or 4) so-called bipolar and unipolar disorders could be forms of the same illness. We will discuss the biology of bipolar depression in the context of these possibilities. For simplicity, we will refer to nonbipolar, recurrent, primary depressions as unipolar depressions.

We define *biology* broadly to include genetic and physiological characteristics, and we will discuss clinical characteristics that can be taken as evidence for underlying biological mechanisms. The basic challenge is to see whether there are biological characteristics that can identify bipolar disorder without relying on a history of mania.

DEPRESSIVE EPISODES IN BIPOLAR DISORDER

Clinical Specificity

The basic depressive syndrome consists of the inhibition of goal-directed and reward-related activity, experienced as anhedonia and anxious pessimism. Biological models for depression have focused largely on the effects of uncontrollable stressors. These models have moderate pharmacological validity but lack evidence of specificity for bipolar disorder (Machado-Vieira et al. 2004; Nestler et al. 2002).

The core depressive or melancholic syndrome appears essentially identical in unipolar and bipolar disorder (Mitchell et al. 1992). On average, bipolar depressive episodes may have more motor retardation and anergy than unipolar depressive episodes (Katz et al. 1982; Kupfer et al. 1974), though not all reports agree with this (Mitchell et al. 1992). Due to substantial overlap with unipolar depression, this characteristic is far from diagnostic (Katz et al. 1982). The same is true for other reported differences between unipolar and bipolar depressions, including the generally, but not uniformly, reported increased incidence of so-called atypical features, including hypersomnia, increased appetite, and rejection sensitivity in bipolar depressions (Benazzi 2003b).

Mixed Depressions

The entire gamut of depressive and manic symptoms, alone or combined, can be present during an exacerbation of bipolar disorder. Mixed mania, in which a manic episode is combined with prominent depressive characteristics, has been studied extensively and is recognized in the DSM-IV-TR. There is also a growing body of literature describing mixed depressions, in which a major depressive episode is usually accompanied by two or more symptoms of mania (Benazzi 2003a). Two manic symptoms were found to be diagnostically overinclusive, present in 78.1% of bipolar and 41.5% of unipolar depressions, while three manic symptoms were present in 46.6% of bipolar and 7.6% of unipolar depressions (Benazzi 2001). It may be possible to improve the definition of mixed depression by prioritizing manic symptoms based on their specificity for mania, as McElroy et al. (1992) did for depressive symptoms in their operational definition of mixed mania. Because anxiety and inner tension are ubiquitous in depressive episodes, agitated depression itself can occur as a mixed state in bipolar disorder (Benazzi et al. 2004) or as an episode of unipolar depression (Katz et al. 1982; Wolff et al. 1985). Clinical differentiation requires 1) identification of other symptoms of mania, such as increased goal-directed activity, grandiosity, hypersexuality, or true racing thoughts that are not depressive or anxious ruminations or obsessions (First et al. 1996); and 2) characterization of the agitation itself, with respect to whether it consists of severe inner tension that is not diagnostic (Frank et al. 2002), or also has a component of driven, goal-directed hyperactivity that would suggest bipolar disorder (Swann et al. 1993). Identifying mixed depressions can require substantial clinical acumen, and the role of mixed depressions, as opposed to mixed manias, has been inadequately studied. Unlike the case with mixed versus nonmixed mania (Swann et al. 1992, 1994), there is little information comparing biological characteristics of mixed versus nonmixed depressions. We reported increased norepinephrine function in predominantly manic mixed states compared with pure depressive episodes (Swann et al. 1994). This review will focus on depressions that do not have prominent mixed features, since they arguably constitute a greater diagnostic challenge.

In summary, bipolar depressions, on average, have more severe motor slowing and atypical features than do nonbipolar depressions, but there is substantial overlap. Some bipolar depressions have demonstrable manic features, but unless these features are present, it is impossible to make the diagnosis of bipolar disorder based on the clinical characteristics of a depressive episode (Abrams and Taylor 1980; Benazzi 1999; Dorz et al. 2003).

STUDIES OF BIOLOGICAL SPECIFICITY

Studies of Neurotransmitter Function

Neurotransmitter function in bipolar and nonbipolar depressions has been investigated using transmitter metabolite levels in body fluids, receptors on peripheral cells, and receptor function using agonist or neuroendocrine challenge techniques. The studies were guided by a series of simple and heuristically useful hypotheses, summarized in Table 2–1. Despite supporting data for each hypothesis, each also had contradictory findings. At a fairly early stage, it was possible to reject hypotheses that major depression, bipolar or otherwise, stemmed from too much or too little of any transmitter (Maas et al. 1991). The second generation of hypotheses held that balances between transmitters, such as norepinephrine versus serotonin (Prange et al. 1974) or norepinephrine (NE) versus acetylcholine (Janowsky et al. 1972), were abnormal. The third generation of hypotheses, logically very close to the first generation, held that second messenger function associated with transmitter receptors was abnormal, usually with increased activity in mania (Lachman and Papolos 1995; Stewart et al. 2001).

Most neurotransmitter studies have focused on norepinephrine. There is a state-dependent elevation of NE function in manic and mixed states (Swann et al. 1987), but there are no reliable changes in NE or its metabolite levels during depression (Koslow et al. 1983). However, NE is apparently metabolized abnormally during depression, with lower relative concentrations of intracellular metabolites, interpreted as consistent with increased, pulsatile release of NE (Maas et al. 1987). This also occurs in mania (Swann et al. 1987). A discriminant analysis of NE and epinephrine metabolite excretion patterns resulted in the D-score, which is generally lowest in bipolar I depression, higher in bipolar II

TABLE 2–1. Classical transmitter hypotheses in bipolar disorder

Hypothesis	Supporting data	References
Norepinephrine high in mania, low in depression	Levels of metabolites in body fluids, responses to treatments, precipitation of episodes, animal models	Bunney et al. 1972
Norepinephrine high in mania and low in depression superimposed on low serotonin in both	Levels of metabolites in body fluids, responses to L-tryptophan	Prange et al. 1974
High norepinephrine and low acetylcholine in mania; opposite in depression	Effects of cholinomimetic drugs on affect, physiological sensitivity to cholinomimetic drugs	Janowsky et al. 1972
Low GABA	GABA levels in body fluids, responses to treatments, animal models	Brambilla et al. 2003

depression, and highest in other depressions (Grossman and Potter 1999; Schatzberg et al. 1989). (The D-score is a mathematical calculation of different amine metabolite levels that "discriminate" between different types of depression [Schatzberg et al. 1989].) This interesting finding is hard to interpret physiologically. The proportion of NE that is metabolized intracellularly rather than excreted unchanged may be easier to interpret physiologically but is reduced in both unipolar and bipolar depressions (Maas et al. 1987).

Regardless of differences in amounts of NE and its metabolites, patients with bipolar disorder appear to have increased reactivity to NE. More so in bipolar than in unipolar depressions, noradrenergic function is more strongly related to mood and psychomotor impairment (Swann et al. 1999), treatment response (Maas et al. 1984), and relationship to stressful events (Swann et al. 1990). Subjects with bipolar disorder have increased sensitivity to subjective effects of stimulants (Anand et al. 2000). Pharmacologically increased NE precipitates mania in subjects with bipolar disorder (Price et al. 1984) and may selectively improve bipolar depression (Osman et al. 1989). Subjects with bipolar disorder have a greater noradrenergic response to orthostasis (Rudorfer et al. 1985) compared with those with unipolar disorder or to controls. A postmortem brain study showed that patients with bipolar disorder had more noradrenergic neurons in the locus coeruleus than did unipolar subjects or controls (Baumann and Bogerts 2001).

Studies of serotonergic function, generally assessed using neuroendocrine or other responses to antagonist, agonist, or precursor infusions, have generally been consistent with reduced functional capacity but have yielded little evidence for specificity between bipolar and unipolar disorders (Price et al. 1991; Sher et al. 2003; Sobczak et al. 2002). Low serotonergic function may be related to potential suicidality in a manner independent of affect or diagnosis (Goodwin and Post 1983; Mann 1999), or the relationship may be stronger in subjects with unipolar depression than in those with bipolar depression (Åsberg 1997). Perhaps the most interesting evidence that there might be a specific relationship between serotonergic function and bipolar disorder is a study that compared relatives of bipolar disorder patients with controls, which found that tryptophan depletion lowered mood and increased impulsivity in relatives of patients with bipolar disorder (Quintin et al. 2001).

Other transmitter-related findings in bipolar depression include increased sensitivity to acetylcholine (Sitaram et al. 1982) and reduced γ-aminobutyric acid (GABA) in body fluids (Brambilla et al. 2003; Petty et al. 1993). Cerebrospinal fluid (CSF) GABA levels in euthymic subjects with bipolar disorder were the same as those in control subjects (Berrettini et al. 1982, 1986); therefore, low GABA levels may be a characteristic of depressive episodes in general. There is also a complex array of endocrine findings, most involving the hypothalamic-pituitary-adrenocortical axis (HPA). Reported HPA abnormalities include increased cortisol excretion with reduced sensitivity to negative feedback regulation, resulting in an increased incidence of dexamethasone nonsuppression in both bipolar and nonbipolar depressions (Stokes et al. 1984). Despite original suggestions that HPA dysfunction was related to a specific type of treatment-responsive depressive episode, there are no reliable or specific clinical differences, other than increased anxiety, between major depressive episodes with and without HPA axis dysfunction (Kocsis et al. 1985). In bipolar disorder, CSF cortisol concentrations and degree of dexamethasone suppression test (DST) nonsuppression are related to depressed mood, especially in mixed states (Swann et al. 1992). In general, the complexity and varying specificity of these transmitter and endocrine findings suggest that they are secondary to some other underlying process.

Table 2–2 summarizes relationships between biological findings and specificity of bipolar depression relative to unipolar depression, and euthymic bipolar control condition. Most effects appear to be related to presence of depression rather than to diagnosis, but there are interesting exceptions. Changes in NE appear state-dependent, but sensitivity to NE appears abnormal regardless of state and differentiates bipolar from unipolar disorder. Most serotonergic abnormalities seem to be similar in bipolar and unipolar disorder, but blunted response to 5-hydroxytryptophan in euthymic subjects and abnormal behavioral responses to tryptophan depletion in relatives of patients with bipolar disorder imply that there may be trait-dependent abnormalities in serotonergic function with some degree of specificity to bipolar disorder. There is relatively little information about other transmitter systems, largely because they are more difficult to study neurochemically, lacking convenient stable metabolites or well-defined ligand infusion procedures.

More recent data suggest that pathophysiology might involve systems related to neuronal adaptations to changes in activity, or second-messenger systems that might underlie the apparent complexity of most biological data. The nitric oxide system is a strategic candidate (Akyol et al. 2004), with one indirect study showing lower plasma arginase and higher nitrite levels in subjects with bipolar disorder compared with control subjects (Van Calker and Belmaker 2000; Yanik et al. 2004). Cell signaling systems, particularly involving inositol and protein kinase C, may be involved in effects of so-called mood-stabilizing drugs (Harwood and Agam 2003). Systems involving membrane lipids, such as the arachidonic acid cascade, may be important and are potentially accessible to brain imaging studies (Rapoport 2001). Biological investigations in bipolar disorder are undergoing a transition from studies driven by pharmacological effects and descriptive data to studies aimed at physiological systems that may underlie depression or the susceptibility to its recurrence.

Physiological Studies

Neurophysiology

Before direct brain imaging studies were available, bipolar depression was studied using electroencephalograms, evoked potentials, and neuropsychological tests. As summarized in Table 2–3, these experiments have produced interesting leads that are consistent with subtle abnormalities in arousal, lateralization, and susceptibility to impulsivity in

TABLE 2–2. Specificity of transmitter–related data in bipolar disorder

Specificity	Transmitter	Finding	Reference
Bipolar, unipolar	Norepinephrine	Metabolism (D-score)	Schatzberg et al. 1989; Grossman and Potter 1999
		Adrenomedullary bipolar<unipolar	Maas et al. 1994
		Response to orthostasis, bipolar>unipolar	Rudorfer et al. 1985
		Sensitivity to NE	Swann et al. 1999
		Increased locus coeruleus cells	Baumann and Bogerts 2001
	Serotonin	Distribution of receptors in postmortem brain	Lopez-Figueroa et al. 2004
	Dopamine	Small basal ganglia in postmortem brain	Baumann and Bogerts 2001
	GABA	Low plasma, CSF GABA	Petty et al. 1993; Brambilla et al. 2003
Bipolar=unipolar	Norepinephrine	Reduced intracellular NE metabolism	Maas et al. 1987
		Metabolite levels	Koslow et al. 1983
		Response to apomorphine	McPherson et al. 2003
		Response to metoclopramide	Joyce et al. 1987
	Serotonin	PET response to fenfluramine	Kegeles et al. 2003
		5-HT-induced Ca++ influx	Kusumi et al. 1994
		Endocrine response to iv tryptophan	Price et al. 1991
		Endocrine response to fenfluramine	Sher et al. 2003
Euthymic bipolar controls	Serotonin	Blunted cortisol response to 5-HTP	Sobczak et al. 2002; Meltzer et al. 1983
		Behavioral response to tryptophan depletion (nonaffected relatives)	Quintin et al. 2001

Note. CSF=cerebrospinal fluid; NE=norepinephrine; PET=positron emission tomography

TABLE 2–3. Some neurophysiological studies in bipolar disorder

Characteristic	Groups compared	Results	Reference
Sensory gating (P50)	Schizophrenia, mania, depression, control	Impairment related to norepinephrine in mania, not in schizophrenia	Adler et al. 1990
Prepulse inhibition	Euthymic bipolar disorder, schizophrenia	Similar impairments	Perry et al. 2001
N1-P2 augmenting	Bipolar vs. unipolar	Bipolar>unipolar	Brocke et al. 2000
	Bipolar vs. nonaffected siblings	Bipolar>sibling	Knott et al. 1985
P300 after oddball stimulus	Schizophrenia, bipolar disorder, control	Decreased amplitude in schizophrenia and bipolar disorder	O'Donnell et al. 2004; Salisbury et al. 1999; Souza et al. 1995
		Prolonged latency in bipolar disorder	Souza et al. 1995
	Bipolar disorder, nonaffected relatives, control	Prolonged latency in bipolar disorder and relatives	Pierson et al. 2000
	Schizophrenia, bipolar, unipolar	Decreased amplitude in subjects with *DISC-1* translocation, regardless of diagnosis	Blackwood and Muir 2004
Laterality	Bipolar, unipolar, control	Loss of right hemispheric dominance	Bruder et al. 1992
	Bipolar, control	Impaired interhemispheric switching	Pettigrew and Miller 1998

bipolar depressive episodes. For example, N1-P2 augmenting was reported to be related to risk for suicidal behavior, regardless of diagnosis (Buchsbaum et al. 1977), and to be inversely proportional to serotonergic function (Brocke et al. 2000; Hegerl et al. 2001); decreased amplitude and delayed onset of P300 was associated with anhedonia (Dubal et al. 2000). One problem in identifying these results is that some of the bipolar depressed patients may have been experiencing mixed episodes, with manic features accounting for some of the findings that differentiated them from nonbipolar depressed patients.

Cation Balance

Abnormalities in arousal or in sensitivity to neurotransmitters may be related to the abnormal regulation of ion distribution (Whybrow and Mendels 1969). Active transport is reduced per sodium pump site in cultured, lymphoblastoid cells from Old Order Amish subjects with bipolar disorder compared with nonaffected relatives or controls (Cherry and Swann 1994). The response of the active transport of sodium to increased sodium influx maintains membrane potential over time in excitable cells, provides the cation gradient that drives uptake processes for neurotransmitters and other compounds and is the major cause of activity-dependent energy utilization (Stahl 1986)—the variable that is measured indirectly by functional brain imaging. This process is diminished in cells from subjects with bipolar disorder (Li and El-Mallakh 2004). Inhibition of the active transport of sodium by ouabain leads to abnormal hippocampal cell excitability (El-Mallakh et al. 2000) and increased motor activity in rats (El-Mallakh et al. 1995, 2003). Genetic studies with genes for subunits of Na,K-ATPase, however, have been negative so far (Li et al. 2000), with the exception of a study suggesting that a specific single nucleotide polymorphism may be overrepresented in the $alpha_3$ isoforms of the alpha subunit in bipolar patients (Mynett-Johnson et al. 1998).

Glial Abnormalities

Glial cells are essential in brain energy metabolism (Schurr et al. 1997b) and are responsible for glutamate clearance. If glial function is diminished, a build up of glutamate could result in overexcitation of neurons (Schurr 2002; Schurr et al. 1997a) with consequent excitotoxicity (Lipton 2004). Several studies have found alterations in glial density in bipolar brain tissue when compared with normal controls: Ongur et al. (1998) found a substantial decrease in glial density in patients with bipolar disorder in the subgenual part of the anterior cingulate cortex (ACC) and the subgenual part of the prefrontal cortex; Chana et al. (2003) showed an increase in neuronal density in the ACC in bipolar disorder; Rajkowska et al. (2001) found a loss of neurons in layer III of the dorsolateral prefrontal cortex; Bowley et al. (2002) reported that glial cell loss in the amygdala was evident only in patients who had not received either lithium or valproate; and Rose et al. (1998) reported that a glia-specific protein, the alpha$_2$ subunit of the sodium potassium ATPase pump, has been found to be reduced in the temporal cortex of bipolar individuals. A subsequent study of temporal tissue found that glial size is reduced in bipolar brains compared with those of normal and depressive controls (Brauch et al., in press).

Relationships Between Biological and Clinical Characteristics

Bipolar and nonbipolar depressions may have similar clinical characteristics, but with different biological mechanisms. For example, impairments of fine motor function can be identical in bipolar and unipolar depressions, but in bipolar depression they are more closely related to noradrenergic function and to severity of the depression (Swann et al. 1999). Similarly, treatment response (Maas et al. 1984) and sensitivity to stressful events (Swann et al. 1990) are more strongly related to norepinephrine in bipolar than in unipolar depressions. In terms of Figure 2–1, these results suggest that clinically similar syndromes have different biological correlates in bipolar and unipolar disorders.

BRAIN IMAGING STUDIES IN BIPOLAR DISORDER

The advent of techniques that can been used to study patterns of neural activity or of receptor function provided a potential advance over previous largely indirect studies of brain function (Dager and Swann 1996). While not always likely to be feasible as general diagnostic techniques, due to expense and the need for sophisticated equipment and data analysis, they have become increasingly widely available and can provide information that can be used to validate peripheral or indirect markers that may be more readily available. Studies using positron emission tomography (PET), single photon emission computed tomography (SPECT), functional and structural magnetic resonance imaging (MRI), and magnetic resonance spectroscopy (MRS) have been carried out in

bipolar depressed subjects, with various comparisons to controls, remitted bipolar subjects, and unipolar depressed subjects (Ketter and
Wang 2002).

Structural Imaging

Results of structural magnetic resonance studies have suggested that
subjects with bipolar disorder were generally more likely than controls
to have white matter hyperintensities, decreased size of the cerebellum,
and increased sulcal and third ventricular volumes (Stoll et al. 2000).
Other studies have not confirmed any specific relationship between bipolar disorder and hyperintensities (Brown et al. 1992; Sassi et al. 2003).
Drevets et al. (1998) reported that subjects with either major depressive
disorder or bipolar disorder had reduced prefrontal cortex gray matter
volume, apparently independent of mood state or treatment. Reduction
in total cortical volume and in volume of the amygdala was reported in
adolescent patients with bipolar disorder, suggesting that the reductions were present early in the course of illness and were not secondary
degenerative changes (DelBello et al. 2004). Hippocampal volume was
reported to be decreased overall in unipolar, but not bipolar, depression (Geuze et al. 2004). In fact, increased right hippocampal volume
was reported to correlate with poor cognitive function in bipolar depressed subjects (Ali et al. 2000). Signal intensity in the corpus callosum was reduced in subjects with bipolar disorder compared with
unipolar disorder or controls (Brambilla et al. 2004), which is consistent
with neuropsychological reports of deficits in interhemispheric switching (Pettigrew and Miller 1998). Overall, these studies suggest that
there are anatomic abnormalities that may exist relatively early in the
course of bipolar disorder, but that their functional and diagnostic sig-
nificances are not fully understood (Kanner 2004).

Functional Imaging

Positron emission tomography and functional magnetic resonance imaging (fMRI) can provide measures related to regional brain activity
(Strakowski et al. 2000). PET studies of glucose metabolism have yielded
results consistent with reduced activity in the prefrontal cortex, which
are consistent with results from nonbipolar depressed subjects (Ketter et
al. 2001; Strakowski et al. 2000). There was also increased activity in the
cerebellar vermis, possibly a trait-related characteristic in bipolar disorder (Ketter et al. 2001). Mood induction studies in subjects with bipolar
disorder (Kruger et al. 2003) found changes in ventral cingulate-corti-

cal-limbic activity that were similar to those found in controls, especially with depressive temperaments (Keightley et al. 2003). A study of anhedonia in bipolar and unipolar depressed subjects revealed that, in both, anhedonia was negatively correlated with 2-deoxyglucose uptake in the insula and claustrum and positively correlated with uptake in the anterior cingulate cortex. Subjects with bipolar disorder had negative correlations between anhedonia and uptake in the dorsolateral prefrontal cortex and the supracallosal cingulate gyrus, while in unipolar depressed subjects anhedonia correlated negatively with uptake into the frontal poles (Dunn et al. 2002). These studies suggest three levels of specificity: subjects with negative affective states regardless of diagnosis (Keightley et al. 2003), depressive subjects regardless of polarity (Dunn et al. 2002; Ketter et al. 2001), and bipolar subjects regardless of affective state (Ketter et al. 2001).

Functional MRI has also been used to study affective and cognitive responsiveness in bipolar disorder. Both bipolar and unipolar disorders appear to be associated with abnormal dorsolateral and ventromedial prefrontal cortex activation (Blumberg et al. 2003; Marvel and Paradiso 2004). Depressed subjects had greater left-ventral prefrontal cortex activation than euthymic subjects, and bipolar subjects had greater rostral left-ventral prefrontal cortical activation than controls in a color-word, emotional, Stroop test (Blumberg et al. 2003). The affective specificity of these responses may differ across diagnoses. In a study of elicited emotions, subjects with bipolar disorder had increased subcortical and ventral, prefrontal, cortical responses to both positive and negative stimuli, compared with unipolar disorder subjects or controls (Lawrence et al. 2004). Another study confirmed that subjects with bipolar disorder differed from controls in responses to both positive and negative stimuli, apparently mobilizing additional subcortical and limbic areas (Malhi et al. 2004).

In Vivo Spectroscopy

Neurochemistry can be studied in vivo using MRS (Moore and Galloway 2002). Proton MRS showed that subjects with bipolar disorder had abnormal choline metabolism, especially in basal ganglia (Strakowski et al. 2000) and the anterior cingulate cortex (Moore et al. 2000). Studies of inositol metabolism, possibly a site of action for lithium, have produced positive (Stoll et al. 2000) and negative (Moore et al. 2000) results. The finding of reduced *N*-acetylaspartate levels in dorsolateral, prefrontal cortex potentially reflects reduced neuronal integrity in that region (Winsberg et al. 2000). Phosphorus MRS suggested the presence of abnormal, frontal, phospholipid metabolism, consistent with earlier metabolic and blood flow studies (Strakowski et al. 2000).

Conclusions

The picture of bipolar depression that is emerging from these brain imaging studies is one in which affective responses are poorly regulated, possibly resulting from failure of the prefrontal cortex to modulate subcortical and temporal signals (Strakowski et al. 2004, 2005). While some abnormalities are present early in the course of illness (DelBello et al. 2004), others may develop as the illness progresses (Strakowski et al. 2004). Imaging studies reveal a complex interaction of diagnostically nonspecific, affective responses superimposed on characteristics more specific for bipolar disorder. Improved characterization of these structural, functional, and metabolic changes will aid in the development of, and increase the need for, a physiological model for the onset and course of bipolar disorder.

BIOLOGY OF BIPOLAR DISORDER IN PATIENTS WITH RECURRENT DEPRESSIONS

Course of Illness

Because the first episode of bipolar disorder is usually depressive, it is important to identify differences between patients with recurrent depressions who eventually had manic episodes and those who continued without manic episodes. Comparisons between these cohorts of identified unipolar and bipolar patients, as well as comparisons between patients with recurrent depressions who did or did not go on to have manic or hypomanic episodes, showed consistently that bipolar disorder has a more recurrent course (Angst et al. 2003; Kessing and Andersen 1999) with earlier onset (Akiskal et al. 1994; Benazzi 2002, 2004; Kessing 1999) and more frequent episodes (Angst et al. 2003; Goldberg and Harrow 2004; Kessing 1999; Kessing and Andersen 1999; Winokur and Wesner 1987). Similarly, rapid cycling can occur in either illness but is substantially more common in bipolar disorder (Wolpert et al. 1990).

These results, combined with the lack of consistent, clinical differences between bipolar and unipolar depressive episodes, support the conclusion that the most salient clinical feature of bipolar disorder is its course of illness, rather than characteristics of individual episodes. In fact, a subgroup of so-called unipolar depressed patients exists who, with high recurrence, lithium sensitivity, and family history, resemble patients with bipolar disorder rather than unipolar disorder (Benazzi 2002, 2003b; Kupfer et al. 1975).

Kindling and sensitization models have been proposed to account for the recurrent course of bipolar disorder (Antelman et al. 1998). These models imply that early episodes would be more likely to be associated with environmental or physiological stressors, with later episodes becoming progressively more autonomous, and that the frequency of episodes would accelerate (Post et al. 1986). In fact, the courses of both bipolar and major depressive disorders, on average, have these general characteristics—for example, both are characterized by early episodes associated with stressful events and later episodes becoming autonomous (Swann et al. 1990). Two large studies of recurrence in well-characterized patients found that bipolar disorder had a higher recurrence rate (Angst et al. 2003; Kessing and Andersen 1999) but that both unipolar and bipolar disorder had increased recurrence rates per episode (9% and 15% respectively) (Kessing and Andersen 1999). These data all suggest that similar mechanisms of recurrence may exist in bipolar and major depressive illness but that in bipolar disorder these mechanisms are, on average, more prominent.

Genetics

Family Studies

Bipolar disorder is highly familial (Gershon et al. 1982). Rate of concordance in monozygotic twins has been reported to range from 47% to 70%, and 5%–10% of first-degree relatives of probands with bipolar disorder also have bipolar disorder (Craddock and Jones 1999). Among offspring of a parent with bipolar disorder, 51% were found to have a psychiatric disorder; risk of bipolar disorder in offspring was increased with early onset of parental illness (Chang et al. 2000). The National Institute of Mental Health (NIMH) Clinical Collaborative Study on the Psychobiology of Depression interviewed 2,225 first-degree relatives of 612 probands, confirming that early onset increased the risk of either unipolar or bipolar disorder in relatives and that the age at onset appeared to be getting earlier in successive generations (Rice et al. 1987). Unipolar disorder is increased in families of subjects with bipolar disorder, so the degree of genetic specificity is not clear (Gershon et al. 1982). Familial and twin studies have not been uniformly successful in demonstrating distinct familial transmission of unipolar and bipolar disorders. A study of an epidemiological sample found an association of mania and major depression in twins, and only a small effect on heritability of major depressive episodes if history of mania was removed, consistent with a continuum model of inheritance for unipolar and bipolar disorders (Karkowski and Kendler 1997). However, in a study of 67 bipolar (30 monozygotic) and 176 unipolar (68 monozygotic) twin pairs, heritability of bipolar disorder was reported to be 85%, with 71% of the genetic risk for mania not shared for depression (McGuffin et al. 2003). A study of 1,578 first-degree relatives of probands with schizophrenia, bipolar disorder, or unipolar disorder found that heritability of affective disorder could be distinguished from schizophrenia but that unipolar disorder could not be clearly distinguished from bipolar disorder.

Candidate Gene Studies

The apparent role of neurotransmitter systems in symptoms of bipolar disorder and in mechanisms of its treatment has led to the investigation of alleles of genes regulating these systems in subjects with bipolar disorder. The results of these studies have been largely negative.

Serotonin. The serotonergic system has been the most extensively studied. A form of the serotonin transporter appears to be related to response to selective serotonin reuptake inhibitors (SSRIs) in either bipolar or unipolar disorder (Lerer and Macciardi 2002; Serretti et al. 2004). Neither tryptophan hydroxylase nor serotonin 1A, 2A, or 2C receptor alleles were related to response to lithium (Serretti et al. 1999, 2000). Incidence of a form of the $5-HT_{2C}$ receptor was reported to be elevated in either unipolar or bipolar disorder (Lerer et al. 2001). Alleles of the $5-HT_{1B}$ (Huang et al. 2003), $5-HT_{2A}$ (Massat et al. 2000; Ni et al. 2002), $5-HT_{5A}$ (Arias et al. 2001), serotonin transporter (Cusin et al. 2001; Mansour et al. 2005), and tryptophan hydroxylase (Cusin et al. 2001) genes were all reported not to distinguish bipolar disorder from unipolar disorder or controls.

Catecholamines. No catecholamine receptor or metabolic enzyme polymorphism has been reported to distinguish bipolar disorder from unipolar disorder or healthy controls. The LL allele of the catechol *O*-methyltransferase (COMT) gene (which has low activity, leading to the potential for reduced extracellular breakdown of catecholamines) was reported to be associated with ultra-rapid cycling in one study (Papolos et al. 1998). The A1 allele of the D_2 dopamine receptor gene was reported to be associated with risk for substance abuse (Noble 2000), and a form of the D_4 receptor was associated with risk of delusions for either unipolar or bipolar disorder (Serretti et al. 1998b). Studies of the NE transporter (Hadley et al. 1995), the alpha$_2$ noradrenergic receptor

(Ohara et al. 1998), the D_3 receptor (Chiaroni et al. 2000), and monoamine oxidase A (MAO-A) (Syagailo et al. 2001) were all negative.

Other transmitters.   Following up on initial theoretical work, research have been disappointed with some recent negative reports regarding GABA-A receptors (Coon et al. 1994; Serretti et al. 1998a), corticotropin-releasing hormone synthesis (Stratakis et al. 1997), and proneurotensin synthesis (Austin et al. 2000).

Physiological systems.   Brain-derived neurotrophic factor (BDNF) is important in neural adaptations to stress and has antidepressant properties in animal models of depression (Hashimoto et al. 2004). A dinucleotide repeat of the BDNF gene was associated with risk for childhood-onset mood disorders (Wood et al. 2003). Results with the val66met allele have been mixed in terms of its ability to distinguish unipolar from bipolar disorder, possibly depending on ethnicity (Hong et al. 2003) or on methods. It did not distinguish bipolar disorder subjects from controls in case-control studies (Nakata et al. 2003; Neves-Pereira et al. 2002; Oswald et al. 2004) or identify subjects with childhood-onset mood disorder (Wood et al. 2003) in case-control studies. In family-based studies, however, the val66met allele was associated with bipolar disorder (Neves-Pereira et al. 2002; Sklar et al. 2002) and childhood-onset bipolar disorder (Geller et al. 2004). This form of BDNF was also associated with early-onset obsessive-compulsive disorder (Hall et al. 2003), which may itself be related to risk for bipolar disorder (Chen and Dilsaver 1995; Thomsen 1992).

   Clock genes have been reported to be associated with increased recurrence in bipolar disorder (Benedetti et al. 2003) and with age at onset (Benedetti et al. 2004). A form of GSK-3-beta may be protective but has a low frequency (Benedetti et al. 2004).

Studies in brain tissue.   Systems of interest can be studied in postmortem brain tissue, by means of quantitative autoradiography and in situ hybridization. There is evidence supporting abnormal regulation of receptor–second messenger signaling, but not in the receptor binding sites themselves for thalamic glutamatergic systems (Clinton et al. 2004). Tantalizing studies reveal reductions in a group of synaptic proteins called *complexins* in limbic areas in schizophrenia and bipolar disorder, but not unipolar disorder (Eastwood and Harrison 2000). Expression of the CREB gene was increased in the amygdala of suicide victims, regardless of diagnosis (Young et al. 2004). A translocation of the DISC-1 gene is associated with reduced P300 amplitude in schizophrenia and bipolar disorder (Blackwood et al. 2001, 2004). Neither COMT (Tunbridge et al. 2004) nor neuropeptide Y (Caberlotto and Hurd 2001) gene expression differed among schizophrenia, bipolar disorder, unipolar disorder, and control samples.

Summary.   The relatively small number of candidate gene alleles that has been studied has not provided much evidence for specific differences between bipolar disorder and either unipolar disorder or schizophrenia. Some characteristics appear to be shared with each. Perhaps the most tantalizing studies are those related to course of illness and to neurophysiological properties. These findings suggest a dimensional pattern of pathophysiology in which bipolar disorder may share some characteristics with schizophrenia and others with unipolar disorder.

Genome Studies

Many potential susceptibility loci have been found, but relatively few findings have been consistently replicated (Craddock and Jones 1999). There appear to be different susceptibility loci associated with paternal or maternal transmission (Cichon et al. 2001a). Significance depends on definition of cases, which ranges from a broad definition that includes all affective disorders to narrow definitions restricted to bipolar I disorder (Cichon et al. 2001b; Segurado et al. 2003). A meta-analysis of 18 data sets found "no strongly significant regions" but did identify promising sites on chromosomes 9, 10, and 14 (Segurado et al. 2003). Similarly, recent studies using NIMH pedigrees, have found "susceptibility genes of modest effect" (Willour et al. 2003; Zandi et al. 2003). A more complete discussion of genome studies is presented in Chapter 3, "Genetics of Bipolar Disorder".

Summary.   Genetic research in bipolar disorder is confirming the complex picture that emerges from clinical research. There appears to be no gene for bipolar disorder, in contrast to illnesses like Huntington's disease. Results of early studies were clouded by inappropriate assumptions of single-gene, dominant inheritance and by problems in identification of cases and controls (Gershon 2000). The most cogent model is that of an oligogenetic disorder, in which clinical characteristics are determined by the combination of several susceptibility genes, each of which may be relatively common (Gershon 2000). Possible domains of susceptibility genes, based on evidence available so far, include onset of illness (Wood et al. 2003), cyclicity (Benedetti et al. 2003), psychosis proneness (Blackwood and Muir 2004), and relative susceptibility to depression or mania (Quitkin et al. 1986).

SUMMARY

Despite substantial progress using brain imaging and genetic techniques, our ability to study the biology of bipolar depression is limited by our imperfect ability to describe the phenotype of bipolar disorder. The presence of past mania or hypomania is not sensitive enough, since depression usually precedes mania. This problem can potentially be addressed by the study of endophenotypes, or characteristics like P300 amplitude or response to stimulants that may represent expression of underlying susceptibility genes (Lenox et al. 2002). Bipolar disorder may share characteristics with schizophrenia or with unipolar disorder, while other features may distinguish it from either illness. This would explain the genetic and clinical overlap between bipolar disorder and both schizophrenia and unipolar disorder, as well as the spectrum-like presentation of affective disorders and schizophrenia.

There are significant clues with regard to specificity, but few findings that are absolute. Depressive episodes associated with bipolar and unipolar disorders can be clinically identical, but depression in bipolar disorder is associated with a stronger interrelationship among affective state, motor function, and noradrenergic function (Swann et al. 1999). The course of illness in bipolar disorder appears to be its most distinctive feature, with earlier onset, more affective lability, and greater susceptibility to recurrence than in unipolar disorder. Yet, these characteristics may represent a continuum where bipolar and unipolar disorders differ quantitatively rather than qualitatively (Angst et al. 2003; Kessing and Andersen 1999; Swann et al. 1990). We suggested a few years ago that the random occurrence of manic episodes might lead to changes in the course of illness that appeared to distinguish unipolar from bipolar disorders (Swann 1997), but there is substantial evidence that frequency of depressive episodes is generally increased before the first manic episode (Akiskal et al. 1994; Winokur and Wesner 1987). Therefore, rather than causing subsequent changes in course of illness, manic episodes may be a random result of increased susceptibility to recurrence of illness, with patients differing in their susceptibility to depression and mania (Quitkin et al. 1986). Finally, the increased susceptibility to stimulants (Anand et al. 2000) and an increased sensitivity to catecholamines (Price et al. 1984; Swann et al. 1990, 1999) suggest a role for behavioral sensitization in bipolar disorder (Post et al. 1986) and the need for a better understanding of the factors that may increase susceptibility to sensitization.

In summary, the convergence of genetic, physiological, and functional imaging studies is moving toward an understanding of mechanisms by which properties determining the course of illness may interact with properties of the depressive syndrome to produce the clinical entity of bipolar depression. We have not yet reached that point. Bipolar and unipolar disorders may be the results of similar underlying processes, but they appear to differ substantially in apparent course and treatment response. The most practical tool for identifying bipolar disorder is still careful characterization of the course of illness.

REFERENCES

Abrams R, Taylor MA: A comparison of unipolar and bipolar depressive illness. Am J Psychiatry 137:1084–1087, 1980

Adler LE, Gerhardt GA, Franks R, et al: Sensory physiology and catecholamines in schizophrenia and mania. Psychiatry Res 31:297–309, 1990

Akiskal HS, Maser JD, Zeller PJ, et al: Switching from 'unipolar' to bipolar II. An 11-year prospective study of clinical and temperamental predictors in 559 patients. Arch Gen Psychiatry 52:114–123, 1994

Akyol O, Zoroglu SS, Armutcu F, et al: Nitric oxide as a physiopathological factor in neuropsychiatric disorders. In Vivo 18:377–390, 2004

Ali SO, Denicoff KD, Altshuler LL, et al: A preliminary study of the relation of neuropsychological performance to neuroanatomic structures in bipolar disorder. Neuropsychiatry Neuropsychol Behav Neurol 13:20–28, 2000

Anand A, Verhoeff P, Seneca N, et al: Brain SPECT imaging of amphetamine-induced dopamine release in euthymic bipolar disorder patients. Am J Psychiatry 157:1108–1114, 2000

Angst J, Gamma A, Sellaro R, et al: Recurrence of bipolar disorders and major depression. A life-long perspective. Eur Arch Psychiatry Clin Neurosci 253:236–240, 2003

Antelman SM, Caggiula AR, Kucinski BJ, et al: The effects of lithium on a potential cycling model of bipolar disorder. Prog Neuropsychopharmacol Biol Psychiatry 22:495–510, 1998

Arias B, Collier DA, Gasto C, et al: Genetic variation in the 5-HT5A receptor gene in patients with bipolar disorder and major depression. Neurosci Lett 303:111–114, 2001

Åsberg M: Neurotransmitters and suicidal behavior: the evidence from cerebrospinal fluid studies. Ann NY Acad Sci 836:158–181, 1997

Austin J, Hoogendoorn B, Buckland P, et al: Association analysis of the pro-neurotensin gene and bipolar disorder. Psychiatr Genet 10:51–54, 2000

Baumann B, Bogerts B: Neuroanatomical studies on bipolar disorder. Br J Psychiatry 41(suppl):s142–s147, 2001

Benazzi F: Bipolar versus unipolar psychotic outpatient depression. J Affect Disord 55:63–66, 1999

Benazzi F: Depressive mixed state: testing different definitions. Psychiatry Clin Neurosci 55:647–652, 2001

Benazzi F: Highly recurrent unipolar may be related to bipolar II. Compr Psychiatry 43:263–268, 2002

Benazzi F: Depressive mixed state: dimensional versus categorical definitions. Prog Neuropsychopharmacol Biol Psychiatry 27:129–134, 2003a

Benazzi F: Is there a link between atypical and early onset "unipolar" depression and bipolar II disorder? Compr Psychiatry 44:102–109, 2003b

Benazzi F: Bipolar II disorder family history using the family history screen: findings and clinical implications. Compr Psychiatry 45:77–82, 2004

Benazzi F, Koukopoulos A, Akiskal HS: Toward a validation of a new definition of agitated depression as a bipolar mixed state (mixed depression). Eur Psychiatry 19:85–90, 2004

Benedetti F, Serretti A, Colombo C, et al: Influence of CLOCK gene polymorphism on circadian mood fluctuation and illness recurrence in bipolar depression. Am J Med Genet 123B:23–26, 2003

Benedetti F, Serretti A, Colombo C, et al: A glycogen synthase kinase 3-beta promoter gene single nucleotide polymorphism is associated with age at onset and response to total sleep deprivation in bipolar depression. Neurosci Lett 368:123–126, 2004

Berrettini WH, Nurnberger JI, Hare T, et al: Plasma and CSF GABA in affective illness. Br J Psychiatry 141:483–487, 1982

Berrettini WH, Nurnberger JI, Hare TA, et al: CSF GABA in euthymic manic-depressive patients and controls. Biol Psychiatry 21:842–844, 1986

Blackwood DH, Muir WJ: Clinical phenotypes associated with DISC1, a candidate gene for schizophrenia. Neurotox Res 6:35–41, 2004

Blackwood DH, Fordyce A, Walker MT, et al: Schizophrenia and affective disorders—cosegregation with a translocation at chromosome 1q42 that directly disrupts brain-expressed genes: clinical and P300 findings in a family. Am J Hum Genet 69:428–433, 2001

Blumberg HP, Leung HC, Skudlarski P, et al: A functional magnetic resonance imaging study of bipolar disorder: state- and trait-related dysfunction in ventral prefrontal cortices. Arch Gen Psychiatry 60:601–609, 2003

Bowley MP, Drevets WC, Ongur D, et al: Low glial numbers in the amygdala in major depressive disorder. Biol Psychiatry 52:404–412, 2002

Brambilla P, Perez J, Barale F, et al: GABAergic dysfunction in mood disorders. Mol Psychiatry 8:721–737, 715, 2003

Brambilla P, Nicoletti M, Sassi RB, et al: Corpus callosum signal intensity in patients with bipolar and unipolar disorder. J Neurol Neurosurg Psychiatry 75:221–225, 2004

Brauch RA, El-Masri MA, Parker JC Jr, et al: Glial cell number and neuron/glial cell ratios in post mortem brains of bipolar individuals. J Affect Disord, in press

Brocke B, Beauducel A, John R, et al: Sensation seeking and affective disorders: characteristics in the intensity dependence of acoustic evoked potentials. Neuropsychobiology 41:24–30, 2000

Brown FW, Lewine RJ, Hudgins PA, et al: White matter hyperintensity signals in psychiatric and nonpsychiatric subjects. Am J Psychiatry 149:620–625, 1992

Bruder GE, Stewart JW, Towey JP, et al: Abnormal cerebral laterality in bipolar depression: convergence of behavioral and brain event-related potential findings. Biol Psychiatry 32:33–47, 1992

Buchsbaum MS, Haier RJ, Murphy DL: Suicide attempts, platelet monoamine oxidase and the average evoked response. Acta Psychiatr Scand 56:69–79, 1977

Bunney WE Jr, Goodwin FK, House KM, et al: The "switch process" in manic-depressive illness: II. Relationship to catecholamines, REM sleep, and drugs. Arch Gen Psychiatry 27:304–309, 1972

Caberlotto L, Hurd YL: Neuropeptide Y Y(1) and Y(2) receptor mRNA expression in the prefrontal cortex of psychiatric subjects. Relationship of Y(2) subtype to suicidal behavior. Neuropsychopharmacology 25:91–97, 2001

Chana G, Landan S, Beasley C, et al: Two dimensional assessment of cytoarchitecture in the anterior cingulate cortex in major depressive disorder, bipolar disorder, and scizophrenia: evidence for decreased neuronal somal size and increased neuronal density. Biol Psychiatry 53:1086–1098, 2003

Chang KD, Steiner H, Ketter TA: Psychiatric phenomenology of child and adolescent bipolar offspring. J Am Acad Child Adolesc Psychiatry 39:453–460, 2000

Chen YW, Dilsaver SC: Comorbidity for obsessive-compulsive disorder in bipolar and unipolar disorders. Psychiatry Res 59:57–64, 1995

Cherry L, Swann AC: Cation transport mediated by Na+,K+-adenosine triphosphatase in lymphoblastoma cells from patients with bipolar I disorder, their relatives, and unrelated control subjects. Psychiatry Res 53:111–118, 1994

Chiaroni P, Azorin JM, Dassa D, et al: Possible involvement of the dopamine D3 receptor locus in subtypes of bipolar affective disorder. Psychiatr Genet 10:43–49, 2000

Cichon S, Schmidt-Wolf G, Schumacher J, et al: A possible susceptibility locus for bipolar affective disorder in chromosomal region 10q25—q26. Mol Psychiatry 6:342–349, 2001a

Cichon S, Schumacher J, Muller DJ, et al: A genome screen for genes predisposing to bipolar affective disorder detects a new susceptibility locus on 8q. Hum Mol Genet 10:2933–2944, 2001b

Clinton SM, Meador-Woodruff JH: Abnormalities of the NMDA receptor and associated intracellular molecules in the thalamus in schizophrenia and bipolar disorder. Neuropsychopharmacology 29:1353–1362, 2004

Coon H, Hicks AA, Bailey ME, et al: Analysis of GABA-A receptor subunit genes in multiplex pedigrees with manic depression. Psychiatr Genet 4:185–191, 1994

Craddock N, Jones I: Genetics of bipolar disorder. J Med Genet 36:585–594, 1999

Cusin C, Serretti A, Lattuada E, et al: Influence of 5-HTTLPR and TPH variants on illness time course in mood disorders. J Psychiatr Res 35:217–223, 2001

Dager SR, Swann AC: Advances in brain metabolism research: toward a moving picture of neural activity. Biol Psychiatry 39:231–233, 1996

DelBello MP, Zimmerman ME, Mills NP, et al: Magnetic resonance imaging analysis of amygdala and other subcortical brain regions in adolescents with bipolar disorder. Bipolar Disord 6:43–52, 2004

Dorz S, Borgherini G, Conforti D, et al: Depression in inpatients: bipolar vs. unipolar. Psychol Reports 92:1031–1039, 2003

Drevets WC, Ongur D, Price JL: Neuroimaging abnormalities in the subgenual prefrontal cortex: implications for the pathophysiology of familial mood disorders. Mol Psychiatry 3:220–221, 1998

Dubal S, Pierson A, Jouvent R: Focused attention in anhedonia: a P3 study. Psychophysiology 37:711–714, 2000

Dunn RT, Kimbrell TA, Ketter TA, et al: Principal components of the Beck Depression Inventory and regional cerebral metabolism in unipolar and bipolar depression. Biol Psychiatry 51:387–399, 2002

Eastwood SL, Harrison PJ: Hippocampal synaptic pathology in schizophrenia, bipolar disorder and major depression: a study of complexin mRNAs. Mol Psychiatry 5:425–432, 2000

El-Mallakh RS, Harrison LT, Li R, et al: An animal model for mania: preliminary results. Prog Neuropsychopharmacol Biol Psychiatry 19:955–962, 1995

El Mallakh RS, Schurr A, Payne RS, Li R: Ouabain induction of cycling of multiple spike responses in hippocampal slices is delayed by lithium. J Psychiatr Res 34:115–120, 2000

El-Mallakh RS, El-Masri MA, Huff MO, et al: Intracerebroventricular administration of ouabain to rats models human mania. Bipolar Disord 5:362–365, 2003

First MB, Spitzer RL, Gibbon M, et al: Structured Clinical Interview for DSM-IV Axis I Disorders, Patient Edition. New York, Biometrics Research Institute, New York State Psychiatric Institute, 1996

Frank E, Rush AJ, Blehar M, et al: Skating to where the puck is going to be: a plan for clinical trials and translation research in mood disorders. Biol Psychiatry 52:631–654, 2002

Geller B, Badner JA, Tillman R, et al: Linkage disequilibrium of the brain-derived neurotrophic factor Val66Met polymorphism in children with a prepubertal and early adolescent bipolar disorder phenotype. Am J Psychiatry 161:1698–1700, 2004

Gershon ES: Bipolar illness and schizophrenia as oligogenic diseases: implications for the future. Biol Psychiatry 47:240–244, 2000

Gershon ES, Hamovit J, Guroff JJ, et al: A family study of schizoaffective, bipolar I, bipolar II, unipolar and normal control probands. Arch Gen Psychiatry 39:1157–1167, 1982

Geuze E, Vermetten E, Bremner JD: MR-based in vivo hippocampal volumetrics, 2: findings in neuropsychiatric disorders. Mol Psychiatry 10:160–184, 2004

Goldberg JF, Harrow M: Consistency of remission and outcome in bipolar and unipolar mood disorders: a 10-year prospective follow-up. J Affect Disord 81:123–131, 2004

Goodwin FK, Post RM: 5-hydroxytryptamine and depression: a model for the interaction of normal variance with pathology. Br J Clin Pharmacol 15:393S–405S, 1983

Grossman F, Potter WZ: Catecholamines in depression: a cumulative study of urinary norepinephrine and its major metabolites in unipolar and bipolar depressed patients versus healthy volunteers at the NIMH. Psychiatry Res 87:21–27, 1999

Hadley D, Hoff M, Holik J, et al: Manic-depression and the norepinephrine transporter gene. Hum Hered 45:165–168, 1995

Hall D, Dhilla A, Charalambous A, et al: Sequence variants of the brain-derived neurotrophic factor (BDNF) gene are strongly associated with obsessive-compulsive disorder. Am J Hum Genet 73:370–376, 2003

Harwood AJ, Agam G: Search for a common mechanism of mood stabilizers. Biochem Pharmacol 66:179–189, 2003

Hashimoto K, Shimizu E, Iyo M: Critical role of brain-derived neurotrophic factor in mood disorders. Brain Res Brain Res Rev 45:104–114, 2004

Hegerl U, Gallinat J, Juckel G: Event-related potentials. Do they reflect central serotonergic neurotransmission and do they predict clinical response to serotonin agonists? J Affect Disord 62:93–100, 2001

Hong CJ, Huo SJ, Yen FC, et al : Association study of a brain-derived neurotrophic-factor genetic polymorphism and mood disorders, age of onset and suicidal behavior. Neuropsychobiology 48:186–189, 2003

Huang YY, Oquendo MA, Friedman JM, et al: Substance abuse disorder and major depression are associated with the human 5-HT1B receptor gene (HTR1B) G861C polymorphism. Neuropsychopharmacology 28:163–169, 2003

Janowsky DS, El-Yousef MK, Davis JM, et al: A cholinergic-adrenergic hypothesis for mania and depression. Lancet 2:632–635, 1972

Kanner AM: Structural MRI changes of the brain in depression. Clin EEG Neurosci 35:46–52, 2004

Karkowski LM, Kendler KS: An examination of the genetic relationship between bipolar and unipolar illness in an epidemiological sample. Psychiatr Genet 7:159–163 1997

Katz MM, Robins E, Croughan J, et al: Behavioral measurement and drug response characteristics of unipolar and bipolar depression. Psychol Med 12:25–36, 1982

Kegeles LS, Malone KM, Slifstein M, et al: Response of cortical metabolic deficits to serotonergic challenge in familial mood disorders. Am J Psychiatry 160:76–82, 2003

Keightley ML, Seminowicz DA, Bagby RM, et al: Personality influences limbic-cortical interactions during sad mood induction. Neuroimage 20:2031–2039, 2003

Kessing LV: The effect of the first manic episode in affective disorder: a case register study of hospitalized episodes. J Affect Disord 53:233–239, 1999

Kessing LV, Andersen PK: The effect of episodes on recurrence of affective disorders: a case register study. J Affect Disord 53:225–231, 1999

Ketter TA, Wang PW: Predictors of treatment response in bipolar disorders: evidence from clinical and brain imaging studies. J Clin Psychiatry 63 (suppl 3):21–25, 2002

Ketter TA, Kimbrell TA, George MS, et al: Effects of mood and subtype on cerebral glucose metabolism in treatment-resistant bipolar disorder. Biol Psychiatry 49:97–109, 2001

Knott V, Waters B, Lapierre Y, et al: Neurophysiological correlates of sibling pairs discordant for bipolar affective disorder. Am J Psychiatry 142:248–250, 1985

Kocsis JH, Davis JM, Katz MM, et al: Depressive behavior and hyperactive adrenocortical function. Am J Psychiatry 142:1291–1298, 1985

Koslow SH, Maas JW, Bowden C, et al: Cerebrospinal fluid and urinary biogenic amines and metabolites in depression, mania, and healthy controls. Arch Gen Psychiatry 40:999–1010, 1983

Kruger S, Seminowicz D, Goldapple K, et al: State and trait influences on mood regulation in bipolar disorder: blood flow differences with an acute mood challenge. Biol Psychiatry 54:1274–1283, 2003

Kupfer DJ, Weiss BL, Foster G, et al: Psychomotor activity in affective states. Arch Gen Psychiatry 30:765–768, 1974

Kupfer DJ, Pickar D, Himmelhoch JM, et al: Are there two types of unipolar depression? Arch Gen Psychiatry 32:866–871, 1975

Kusumi I, Koyama T, Yamashita I: Serotonin-induced platelet intracellular calcium mobilization in depressed patients. Psychopharmacol 113:322–327, 1994

Lachman HM, Papolos DF: A molecular model for bipolar affective disorder. Med Hypotheses 45:255–264, 1995

Lawrence NS, Williams AM, Surguladze S, et al: Subcortical and ventral prefrontal cortical neural responses to facial expressions distinguish patients with bipolar disorder and major depression. Biol Psychiatry 55:578–587, 2004

Lenox RH, Gould TD, Manji HK: Endophenotypes in bipolar disorder. Am J Med Genet 114:391–406, 2002

Lerer B, Macciardi F: Pharmacogenetics of antidepressant and mood-stabilizing drugs: a review of candidate-gene studies and future research directions. Int J Neuropsychopharmacol 5:255–275, 2002

Lerer B, Macciardi F, Segman RH, et al: Variability of 5-HT2C receptor cys23ser polymorphism among European populations and vulnerability to affective disorder. Mol Psychiatry 6:579–585, 2001

Li R, El Mallakh RS: Differential response of bipolar and normal control lymphoblastoid cell sodium pump to ethacrynic acid. J Affect Disord 80:11–17, 2004

Li R, El Mallakh RS, Herman MM, et al: Trinucleotide repeat expansion in the beta1 subunit of the sodium pump in manic-depression illness: a negative study. J Affect Disord 60:131–136, 2000

Lipton SA: Failures and successes of NMDA receptor antagonists: molecular basis for the use of open-channel blockers like memantine in the treatment of acute and chronic neurologic insults. NeuroRx 1:101–110, 2004

Lopez-Figueroa AL, Norton CS, Lopez-Figueroa MO, et al: Serotonin 5-HT1A, 5-HT1B, and 5-HT2A receptor mRNA expression in subjects with major depression, bipolar disorder, and schizophrenia. Biol Psychiatry 55:225–233, 2004

Maas JW, Koslow SH, Katz MM, et al: Pretreatment neurotransmitter metabolite levels and response to tricyclic antidepressant drugs. Am J Psychiatry 141:1159–1171, 1984

Maas JW, Koslow SH, Davis JM, et al: Catecholamine metabolism and disposition in healthy and depressed subjects. Arch Gen Psychiatry 44:337–344, 1987

Maas JW, Katz MM, Frazer A, et al: Current evidence regarding biological hypotheses of depression and accompanying pathophysiological processes: a critique and synthesis of results using clinical and basic research results. Integr Psychiatry 7:155–161, 1991

Maas JW, Katz MM, Koslow SH, et al: Adrenomedullary function in depressed patients. J Psychiatr Res 28:357–367, 1994

Machado-Vieira R, Kapczinski F, Soares JC: Perspectives for the development of animal models of bipolar disorder. Prog Neuro-Psychopharmacol Biol Psychiatry 28:209–224, 2004

MacQueen GM, Young LT, Robb JC, et al: Effect of number of episodes on well-being and functioning of patients with bipolar disorder. Acta Psychiatr Scand 101:374–381, 2000

Malhi GS, Lagopoulos J, Ward PB, et al: Cognitive generation of affect in bipolar depression: an fMRI study. Eur J Neurosci 19:741–754, 2004

Mann JJ: Role of the serotonergic system in the pathogenesis of major depression and suicidal behavior. Neuropsychopharmacology 21:99S–105S, 1999

Mansour HA, Talkowski ME, Wood J, et al: Serotonin gene polymorphisms and bipolar I disorder: focus on the serotonin transporter. Ann Med 37:590–602, 2005

Marvel CL, Paradiso S: Cognitive and neurological impairment in mood disorders. Psychiatr Clin North Am 27:19–36, 2004

Massat I, Souery D, Lipp O, et al: A European multicenter association study of HTR2A receptor polymorphism in bipolar affective disorder. Am J Med Genet 96:136–140, 2000

McElroy SL, Keck PE Jr, Pope HG Jr, et al: Clinical and research implications of the diagnosis of dysphoric or mixed mania or hypomania. Am J Psychiatry 149:1633–1644, 1992

McGuffin P, Rijsdijk F, Andrew M, et al: The heritability of bipolar affective disorder and the genetic relationship to unipolar depression. Arch Gen Psychiatry 60:497–502, 2003

McPherson H, Walsh A, Silverstone T: Growth hormone and prolactin response to apomorphine in bipolar and unipolar depression. J Affect Disord 76:121–125, 2003

Meltzer HY, Uberkoman-Wiita B, Robertson A, et al: Enhanced serum cortisol response to 5-hydroxytryptophan in depression and mania. Life Sci 33:2541–2549, 1983

Mitchell P, Parker G, Jamieson K, et al: Are there any differences between bipolar and unipolar melancholia? J Affect Disord 25:97–105, 1992

Moore GJ, Galloway MP: Magnetic resonance spectroscopy: neurochemistry and treatment effects in affective disorders. Psychopharmacol Bull 36:5–23, 2002

Moore CM, Breeze JL, Gruber SA, et al: Choline, myo-inositol and mood in bipolar disorder: a proton magnetic resonance spectroscopic imaging study of the anterior cingulate cortex. Bipolar Disord 2:207–216, 2000

Mynett-Johnson L, Murphy V, McCormack J, et al: Evidence for an allelic association between bipolar disorder and a Na+,K+ adenosine triphosphatase alpha subunit gene (ATP1A3). Biol Psychiatry 44:47–51, 1998

Nakata K, Ujike H, Sakai A, et al: Association study of the brain-derived neurotrophic factor (BDNF) gene with bipolar disorder. Neurosci Lett 337:17–20, 2003

Nestler EJ, Gould E, Manji H, et al: Preclinical models: status of basic research in depression. Biol Psychiatry 52:503–528, 2002

Neves-Pereira M, Mundo E, Muglia P, et al: The brain-derived neurotrophic factor gene confers susceptibility to bipolar disorder: evidence from a family based association study. Am J Hum Genet 71:651–655, 2002

Ni X, Trakalo JM, Mundo E, et al: Family based association study of the serotonin-2A receptor gene (5-HT$_{2A}$) and bipolar disorder. Neuromolecular Med 2:251–259, 2002

Noble EP: Addiction and its reward process through polymorphisms of the D2 dopamine receptor gene: a review. Eur Psychiatry 15:79–89, 2000

O'Donnell BF, Vohs JL, Hetrick WP, et al: Auditory event-related potential abnormalities in bipolar disorder and schizophrenia. Int J Psychophysiol 53:45–55, 2004

Ohara K, Nagai M, Tani K, et al: Polymorphism in the promoter region of the alpha 2A adrenergic receptor gene and mood disorders. Neuroreport 9:1291–1294, 1998

Ongur P, Drevets WC, Price JL: Glial reduction in the subgenual prefrontal cortex in mood disorders. Proc Natl Acad Sci USA 95:13290–13295, 1998

Osman OT, Rudorfer MV, Potter WZ: Idazoxan: a selective α_2 antagonist and effective sustained antidepressant in two bipolar depressed patients. Arch Gen Psychiatry 46:958–959, 1989

Oswald P, Del Favero J, Massat I, et al: Non-replication of the brain-derived neurotrophic factor (BDNF) association in bipolar affective disorder: a Belgian patient-control study. Am J Med Genet 129B:34–35, 2004

Papolos DF, Veit S, Faedda GL, et al: Ultra-ultra rapid cycling bipolar disorder is associated with the low activity catecholamine-O-methyltransferase allele. Mol Psychiatry 3:346–349, 1998

Perry W, Minassian A, Feifel D, et al: Sensorimotor gating deficits in bipolar disorder patients with acute psychotic mania. Biol Psychiatry 50:418–424, 2001

Perugi G, Micheli C, Akiskal HS, et al: Polarity of the first episode, clinical characteristics, and course of manic depressive illness: a systematic retrospective investigation of 320 bipolar I patients. Compr Psychiatry 41:13–18, 2000

Pettigrew JD, Miller SM: A 'sticky' interhemispheric switch in bipolar disorder? Proc R Soc Lond B Biol Sci 265:2141–2148, 1998

Petty F, Kramer GL, Fulton M, et al: Low plasma GABA is a trait-like marker for bipolar illness. Neuropsychopharmacology 9:125–132, 1993

Pierson A, Jouvent R, Quintin P, et al: Information processing deficits in relatives of manic depressive patients. Psychol Med 30:545–555, 2000

Post RM, Rubinow DR, Ballenger JC: Conditioning and sensitization in the longitudinal course of affective illness. Br J Psychiatry 149:191–201, 1986

Post RM, Denicoff KD, Leverich GS, et al: Morbidity in 258 bipolar outpatients followed for 1 year with daily prospective ratings on the NIMH life chart method. J Clin Psychiatry 64:680–690, 2003

Prange AJ, Wilson JC, Lynn CW, et al: L-tryptophan in mania: contribution to a permissive hypothesis of affective disorders. Arch Gen Psychiatry 30:56–62, 1974

Price LH, Charney DS, Heninger GR: Three cases of manic symptoms following yohimbine administration. Am J Psychiatry 141:1267–1268, 1984

Price LH, Charney DS, Delgado PL, et al: Serotonin function and depression: neuroendocrine and mood responses to intravenous L-tryptophan in depressed patients and healthy comparison subjects. Am J Psychiatry 148:1518–1525, 1991

Quintin P, Benkelfat C, Launay JM, et al: Clinical and neurochemical effect of acute tryptophan depletion in unaffected relatives of patients with bipolar affective disorder. Biol Psychiatry 50:184–190, 2001

Quitkin FM, Rabkin JG, Prien RF: Bipolar disorder: are there manic-prone and depressive-prone forms? J Clin Psychopharmacol 6:167–172, 1986

Rajkowska G, Halaris A, Selemon LD: Reductions in neuronal and glial density characterize the dorsolateral prefrontal cortex in bipolar disorder. Biol Psychiatry 49:741–752, 2001

Rapoport SI: In vivo fatty acid incorporation into brain phosholipids in relation to plasma availability, signal transduction and membrane remodeling. J Mol Neurosci 16:243–261, 2001

Rice J, Reich T, Andreasen NC, et al: The familial transmission of bipolar illness. Arch Gen Psychiatry 44:441–447, 1987

Rose AM, Mellett BJ, Valdes R Jr, et al: Alpha2 isoform of the Na,K-ATPase is reduced in temporal cortex of bipolar individuals. Biol Psychiatry 44:892–897, 1998

Rudorfer MV, Ross RJ, Linnoila M, et al: Exaggerated orthostatic responsivity of plasma norepinephrine in depression. Arch Gen Psychiatry 42:1186–1192, 1985

Salisbury DF, Shenton ME, McCarley RW: P300 topography differs in schizophrenia and manic psychosis. Biol Psychiatry 45:98–106, 1999

Sassi RB, Brambilla P, Nicoletti M, et al: White matter hyperintensities in bipolar and unipolar patients with relatively mild-to-moderate illness severity. J Affect Disord 77:237–245, 2003

Schatzberg AF, Samson JA, Bloomingdale KL, et al: Toward a biochemical classification of depressive disorders. X. Urinary catecholamines, their metabolites, and D-type scores in subgroups of depressive disorders. Arch Gen Psychiatry 46:260–268, 1989; erratum Arch Gen Psychiatry 46:860, 1989

Schurr A: Energy metabolism, stress hormones and neural recovery from cerebral ischemia/hypoxia. Neurochem Int 41:1–8, 2002

Schurr A, Payne R, Miller J, et al: Brain lactate, not glucose, fuels the recovery of synaptic function from hypoxia upon reoxygenation: an in vitro study. Brain Res 744:105–111, 1997a

Schurr A, Payne R, Miller J, et al: Glia are the main source of lactate utilized by neurons for recovery of function posthypoxia. Brain Res 774:221–224, 1997b

Segurado R, Detera-Wadleigh SD, Levinson DF, et al: Genome scan meta-analysis of schizophrenia and bipolar disorder, part III: bipolar disorder. Am J Hum Genet 73:49–62, 2003

Serretti A, Macciardi F, Cusin C, et al: Dopamine receptor D4 gene is associated with delusional symptomatology in mood disorders. Psychiatry Res 80:129–136, 1998a

Serretti A, Macciardi F, Cusin C, et al: GABAA alpha-1 subunit gene not associated with depressive symptomatology in mood disorders. Psychiatr Genet 8:251–254, 1998b

Serretti A, Lilli R, Lorenzi C, et al: Tryptophan hydroxylase gene and response to lithium prophylaxis in mood disorders. J Psychiatr Res 33:371–377, 1999

Serretti A, Lorenzi C, Lilli R, et al: Serotonin receptor 2A, 2C, 1A genes and response to lithium prophylaxis in mood disorders. J Psychiatr Res 34:89–98, 2000

Serretti A, Cusin C, Rossini D, et al: Further evidence of a combined effect of SERTPR and TPH on SSRIs response in mood disorders. Am J Med Genet 129B:36–40, 2004

Sher L, Oquendo MA, Li S, et al: Prolactin response to fenfluramine administration in patients with unipolar and bipolar depression and healthy controls. Psychoneuroendocrinology 28:559–573, 2003

Sitaram N, Nurnberger JI Jr, Gershon ES, et al: Cholinergic regulation of mood and REM sleep: potential model and marker of vulnerability to affective disorder. Am J Psychiatry 139:571–576, 1982

Sklar P, Gabriel SB, McInnis MG, et al: Family based association study of 76 candidate genes in bipolar disorder: BDNF is a potential risk locus. Brain-derived neutrophic factor. Mol Psychiatry 7:579–593, 2002

Sobczak S, Honig A, van Duinen MA, et al: Serotonergic dysregulation in bipolar disorders: a literature review of serotonergic challenge studies. Bipolar Disord 4:347–356, 2002

Souza VB, Muir WJ, Walker MT, et al: Auditory P300 event-related potentials and neuropsychological performance in schizophrenia and bipolar affective disorder. Biol Psychiatry 37:300–310, 1995

Stahl WL: The Na,K-ATPase of nervous tissue. Neurochem Int 8:449–476, 1986

Stewart RJ, Chen B, Dowlatshahi D, et al: Abnormalities in the cAMP signaling pathway in post-mortem brain tissue from the Stanley Neuropathology Consortium. Brain Res Bull 55:625–629, 2001

Stokes PE, Stoll PM, Koslow SH, et al: Pretreatment DST and hypothalamic-pituitary-adrenocortical function in depressed patients and comparison groups. Arch Gen Psychiatry 41:257–267, 1984

Stoll AL, Renshaw PF, Yurgelun-Todd DA, et al: Neuroimaging in bipolar disorder: what have we learned? Biol Psychiatry 48:505–517, 2000

Strakowski SM, DelBello MP, Adler C, et al: Neuroimaging in bipolar disorder. Bipolar Disord 2:148–164, 2000

Strakowski SM, Adler CM, Holland SK, et al: A preliminary fMRI study of sustained attention in euthymic, unmedicated bipolar disorder. Nueropsychopharmacol 29:1734–1740, 2004

Strakowski SM, DelBello MP, Adler CM: The functional neuroanatomy of bipolar disorder: a review of neuroimaging findings. Mol Psychiatry 10:105–116, 2005

Stratakis CA, Sarlis NJ, Berrettini WH, et al: Lack of linkage between the corticotropin-releasing hormone (CRH) gene and bipolar affective disorder. Mol Psychiatry 2:483–485, 1997

Swann AC: Is bipolar depression a specific biological entity? In Bipolar Disorder: Biological Models and Their Clinical Applications. Edited by Young LT, Joffe RT. New York, Marcel Dekker, 1997, pp 255–285

Swann AC, Koslow SH, Katz MM, et al: Lithium carbonate treatment of mania. Cerebrospinal fluid and urinary monoamine metabolites and treatment outcome. Arch Gen Psychiatry 44:345–354, 1987

Swann AC, Secunda SK, Stokes PE, et al: Stress, depression, and mania: relationship between perceived role of stressful events and clinical and biochemical characteristics. Acta Psychiatr Scand 81:389–397, 1990

Swann AC, Stokes PE, Casper R, et al: Hypothalamic-pituitary-adrenocortical function in mixed and pure mania. Acta Psychiatr Scand 85:270–274, 1992

Swann AC, Secunda SK, Katz MM, et al: Specificity of mixed affective states: clinical comparison of mixed mania and agitated depression. J Affective Disord 28:81–89, 1993

Swann AC, Stokes PE, Secunda S, et al: Depressive mania vs agitated depression: biogenic amine and hypothalamic-pituitary-adrenocortical function. Biol Psychiatry 35:803–813, 1994

Swann AC, Katz MM, Bowden CL, et al: Psychomotor performance and monoamine function in bipolar and unipolar affective disorders. Biol Psychiatry 45:979–988, 1999

Syagailo YV, Stober G, Grassle M, et al: Association analysis of the functional monoamine oxidase A gene promoter polymorphism in psychiatric disorders. Am J Med Genet 105:168–171, 2001

Thomsen PH: Obsessive-compulsive disorder in adolescence. Differential diagnostic considerations in relation to schizophrenia and manic-depressive disorder: a comparison of phenomenology and sociodemographic characteristics. Psychopathology 25:301–310, 1992

Tunbridge E, Burnet PW, Sodhi MS, et al: Catechol-O-methyltransferase (COMT) and proline dehydrogenase (PRODH) mRNAs in the dorsolateral prefrontal cortex in schizophrenia, bipolar disorder, and major depression. Synapse 51:112–118, 2004

Van Calker D, Belmaker RH: The high affinity inositol transport system—implications for the pathophysiology and treatment of bipolar disorder. Bipolar Disord 2:102–107, 2000

Whybrow P, Mendels J: Toward a biology of depression: some suggestions from neurophysiology. Am J Psychiatry 125:45–54, 1969

Willour VL, Zandi PP, Huo Y, et al: Genome scan of the fifty-six bipolar pedigrees from the NIMH genetics initiative replication sample: chromosomes 4, 7, 9, 18, 19, 20, and 21. Am J Med Genet 121B:21–27, 2003

Winokur G, Wesner R. From unipolar depression to bipolar illness: 29 who changed. Acta Psychiatr Scand 76:59–63, 1987

Winsberg ME, Sachs N, Tate DL, et al: Decreased dorsolateral prefrontal N-acetyl aspartate in bipolar disorder. Biol Psychiatry 47:475–481, 2000

Wolff EAI, Putnam FW, Post RM: Motor activity and affective illness: the relationship of amplitude and temporal distribution to changes in affective state. Arch Gen Psychiatry 42:288–294, 1985

Wolpert EA, Goldberg JF, Harrow M: Rapid-cycling in unipolar and bipolar affective disorders. Am J Psychiatry 147:725–728, 1990

Wood SJ, Berger G, Velakoulis D, et al: Proton magnetic resonance spectroscopy in first episode psychosis and ultra high-risk individuals. Schizophr Bull 29:831–843, 2003

Yanik M, Vural H, Tutkun H, et al: The role of the arginine-nitric oxide pathway in the pathogenesis of bipolar affective disorder. Eur Arch Psychiatry Clin Neurosci 254:43–47, 2004

Young LT, Bezchlibnyk YB, Chen B, et al: Amygdala cyclic adenosine mono-
    phosphate response element binding protein phosphorylation in patients
    with mood disorders: effects of diagnosis, suicide, and drug treatment. Biol
    Psychiatry 55:570–577, 2004
Zandi PP, Willour VL, Huo Y, et al: Genome scan of a second wave of NIMH ge-
    netics initiative bipolar pedigrees: chromosomes 2, 11, 13, 14, and X. Am
    J Med Genet 119B:69–76, 2003

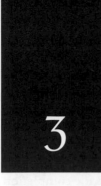

GENETICS OF
BIPOLAR DISORDER

Elizabeth P. Hayden, Ph.D.
John I. Nurnberger Jr., M.D., Ph.D.

BIPOLAR DISORDER IS A severe condition typically characterized by manic and depressive episodes, affecting about 0.5%–1% of the population in its most narrowly defined form. Often seen in conjunction with suicidality, psychiatric comorbidity, and pronounced impairment in psychosocial functioning, bipolar disorder exacts a great toll on patients and their families. Even with adequate treatment with a mood stabilizer, one-third of bipolar patients relapse within 3 years (Keller et al. 1992), and annual costs for adult Americans with the disorder were estimated at $45 billion in 1991 (Wyatt and Henter 1995). Bipolar disorder has been ranked as the sixth leading cause of disability worldwide (Murray and Lopez 1996). As befitting an illness with such harmful sequelae, there is great interest in refining our understanding of the etiology of the disease. Research from twin and adoption studies consistently indicates a strong and compelling influence of genetics on bipolar disorder. Several twin studies have shown a markedly elevated risk of bipolar disorder in monozygotic twins compared with dizygotic twins

Portions of this work were supported by AA07462, MH059545, and an unnumbered grant from the Indiana Division of Mental Health.

(e.g., Bertelsen et al. 1977; Cardno et al. 1999; Kendler et al. 1993b). Adoption studies also testify to the importance of genetic factors in bipolar disorder: the disorder is more common among the biological parents than among the adoptive parents of bipolar adoptees (Mendelwicz and Rainer 1977), and Wender et al. (1986) reported that biological relatives of adopted bipolar probands show elevated rates of a variety of psychiatric illnesses and suicide completion.

It is well established that the more severe forms of affective illness, such as bipolar disorder, run in families and appear to be highly heritable. Examining pedigrees of patients with affective disorders suggests a genetic mode of inheritance incompatible with a single-gene explanation, and extant research suggests both shared and unique genetic variance within the family of affective disorders. Both unipolar and bipolar depression are seen in families of bipolar probands, whereas primarily unipolar depression is seen in families of unipolar-depressed probands, indicating a shared genetic susceptibility between some forms of unipolar and bipolar illness. Similarly, although bipolar II disorder (depression accompanied by hypomania) appears to be genetically related to both bipolar disorder and unipolar depression, there is some evidence for higher rates of bipolar II illness in the families of bipolar II probands (Gershon et al. 1987), which suggests that some genetic influences are unique to bipolar II illness.

Despite consistent evidence from twin, adoption, and family studies supporting the role of genes in bipolar disorder, the precise molecular bases for the disorder appear complex and are poorly understood. Although some chromosomal regions have more consistent support than others, to date no specific gene has been identified that is known to contribute incontrovertibly to the etiology of bipolar disorder. In an attempt to consolidate current knowledge of the genetic bases for bipolar illness, we will here summarize findings from linkage and association studies with an emphasis on papers published since 1999. In determining which studies to include, we generally follow cutoffs recommended by Lander and Kruglyak (1995) for significant and suggestive logarithm of odds (LOD) scores, except in instances where multiple studies implicate the same region. In such cases, we may also include studies reporting LOD scores that approach these cutoffs. We will then consider a variety of strategies for future research on the genetic bases for bipolar disorder.

HIGH-INDEX ASSOCIATIONS

Certain sections of the human chromosome have been more closely associated with bipolar illness than others. These high-index associations have been replicated and may identify important candidate genes. Despite these high-index associations, no specific genes have been definitively identified as contributing to the risk of developing bipolar illness or protecting against its development, or with any of the treatment or course variables associated with this disorder.

Chromosome 4

Significant linkage to chromosome 4p was initially reported by Blackwood and colleagues in a large Scottish pedigree (Blackwood et al. 1996). Detera-Wadleigh et al. (1999) also reported linkage evidence for 4p16–p14. Suggestive linkage has also been reported to chromosome 4q35 by Adams et al. (1998) in an Australian pedigree. Several studies have detected linkage signals on various regions of the chromosome. McInnis et al. (2003b) examined a sample of 65 bipolar probands from inpatient and outpatient clinics in Maryland and Iowa and their families. The Research Diagnostic Criteria (RDC) were used for diagnoses, and the Center for Inherited Disease Research genotyped the majority of the pedigrees for markers. Using GENEHUNTER-PLUS (Kong and Cox 1997), nonparametric, genome-wide linkage analysis revealed a weak linkage signal around the *D4S1629* marker (LOD=1.9 for a broad disease model) on 4q32. Badenhop et al. (2003) examined a 55-pedigree sample containing 674 British and Irish individuals available for analyses. Diagnoses were made according to the RDC. Twenty-nine microsatellite markers on chromosome 4q35 were used, and two-point parametric LOD score analyses were conducted using ANALYZE (Hiekkalina et al. 2005). Several markers in this region showed suggestive evidence for linkage, including *D4S3051* (LOD=2.32), *D4S426* (LOD=2.49), and *D4S1652* (LOD=3.19), all under a broad disease model. In the study described earlier of Liu and colleagues (2003), *D4S1625* at 4q31 gave a suggestive two-point LOD score of 3.16 under a dominant model, using a broadly defined disease phenotype.

Linkage findings to 4p16, along with findings that suggest psychiatric symptoms are associated with Wolfram's disease (Nanko et al. 1992), have led to the hypothesis that the Wolfram gene (*WFS1*/wolframin) may be a plausible candidate gene for bipolar disorder. With regard to association studies of this region, Kato et al. (2003) examined the association between mutations and mRNA expression of *WFS1* and bipolar disorder in a Japanese sample of 184 unrelated patients with bipolar disorders and 207 unrelated control subjects. The authors found no significant differences in mutations or expression of *WFS1* mRNA between the groups, suggesting a lack of importance of this gene in bipolar illness.

Chromosome 11

Chromosome 11 has been of interest to investigators since the first indication of linkage in an Old Order Amish kindred. Recent association and linkage studies continue to suggest that chromosome 11 may play a role in bipolar disorder. As part of the National Institute of Mental Health (NIMH) Genetics Initiative on bipolar disorder, Zandi and colleagues (2003) scanned chromosomes 2, 11, 13, 14, and X in 56 families of 354 individuals. Microsatellite markers were used, and multipoint parametric and nonparametric analyses were conducted by using GENE-HUNTER-PLUS and X-GENEHUNTER v1.3 (Kong and Cox 1997). The authors reported a peak nonparametric linkage score of 2.96 at the marker *D11S1923*. Parametric analysis revealed a suggestive heterogeneity LOD score of 2.0 near this same marker under a dominant, intermediate disease model. They were also able to estimate that a likely location of this gene is in close proximity to the tyrosine hydroxylase (*TH*) gene, the rate-limiting enzyme in the synthesis of catecholamines, which may play a role in the pathophysiology of bipolar disorder. *TH* has previously been reported to be a candidate by Mallet and colleagues (e.g., Meloni et al. 1995) and may have an association with major depression, particularly with a polymorphism at intron 7 (Gizatullin et al. 2005).

Muglia and colleagues (2002) investigated the role of the dopamine D_4 receptor (*DRD4*) and *TH* genes (both located on 11p) in bipolar disorder in a sample of 154 patients with a diagnosis of bipolar I or bipolar II disorder, schizoaffective disorder, bipolar type (SABP), or bipolar disorder not otherwise specified, and their biological parents in a sample of 145 nuclear families. The sample was Canadian and predominantly Caucasian. They did not find biases in *TH* allele transmission. Similarly, an association could not be documented in a Taiwanese sample (Lai et al. 2005). However, excessive transmission of the *DRD4* 4-repeat alleles was detected, whereas the 2-repeat allele was transmitted at reduced rates, leading Muglia et al. (2002) to suggest that this allele may provide protection from risk for bipolar disorder. Their analyses indicated a parent-of-origin effect, in that transmission of both the 4-repeat and 2-repeat alleles was associated with the maternal meiosis.

Sklar et al. (2002) examined the association between a variety of candidate genes and bipolar disorder by genotyping single nucleotide polymorphic markers (SNPs) in these genes in 136 patient-parent triads. Recruited by investigators at Johns Hopkins University, these families from the same sample as McInnis et al. (2003b) were recruited from inpatient and outpatient clinics in Maryland and Iowa and were diagnosed following the RDC. Probands had a diagnosis of either bipolar I or bipolar II disorder or schizoaffective mania. An association between bipolar disorder and SNPs in the brain-derived neurotrophic factor gene (*BDNF*), which maps to chromosome 11p13–15, was found. Sklar et al. (2002) confirmed this association in two independent samples of bipolar patients (although it appears that multiple family members were treated as independent cases). In the replication samples, excess transmission of the valine allele of amino acid 66 of *BDNF* was observed. Further evidence for the role of *BDNF* in bipolar disorder was reported by Neves-Pereira et al. (2002), although negative results have been reported as well (Nakata et al. 2003). Although the functional significance of *BDNF* in bipolar disorder is unclear, Sklar et al. (2002) noted that animal models suggest *BDNF* may be involved in mood regulation, and BDNF levels are increased by lithium treatment (Einat et al. 2003).

Authors have suggested that dysregulation of the dopaminergic system could explain the radical mood shifts that characterize bipolar disorder (Willner et al. 1991, 1992), making the genes involved in this system plausible candidates. Massat et al. (2002b) investigated the role of the dopamine D_2 receptor gene (*DRD2*) at 11q22.2–22.3 in a multisite European study of affective disorders. A total of 469 bipolar patients and 524 matched controls were genotyped for the *DRD2* marker. An association between bipolar disorder and overexpression of the 5–5 genotype and a higher frequency of allele 5 was found in bipolar patients.

Nearby on 11q23.1, polymorphisms of the neural cell adhesion molecule 1 gene (*NCAM1*) were found to be nominally associated with bipolar disorder in a Japanese sample of 151 patients, compared with 357 control subjects (Arai et al. 2004). *NCAM1* is involved in an array of neurodevelopmental processes that may contribute to bipolar disorder susceptibility if disrupted, but that may be more important in the pathophysiology of schizophrenia (Poltorak et al. 1995).

Chromosome 12

Linkage to chromosome 12 was reported by Craddock and colleagues (1999) in a family in which major affective disorder was co-segregating with Darier's disease. Morissette and colleagues (1999) examined a very large French Canadian pedigree, finding evidence for linkage (several LOD scores >1.5) to chromosome 12q23–q24 in some, but not all, branches of the pedigree. Analysis of a second, smaller pedigree from the same geographic region also appeared to support evidence of a locus on chromosome 12. Additionally, Barden (2003) reported a significant association to an unnamed gene around the 12q23–24 region, using haplotype analysis. Curtis et al. (2003) reported that a dominant model including cases of unipolar depression obtained a suggestive four-point LOD score of 2.8 for the marker *D12S342*, which is near the Darier's disease region. In two families, Ewald et al. (2002b) reported a significant genome-wide multipoint parametric LOD score of 3.63 at *D12S1639*, further supporting the notion that this region contains susceptibility genes for bipolar disorder. However, other evidence suggests that while regions near the Darier's disease gene may confer bipolar vulnerability, it may not be the Darier's disease gene itself that does so (Jacobsen et al. 2001; Jones et al. 2002).

Chromosome 16

After finding suggestive linkage signals at marker *D16S2619* in both the original and replication samples from the NIMH Genetics Initiative, Dick et al. (2002) examined the combined samples for additional evidence of linkage. Using nonparametric affected relative pair analysis, they identified a region containing four markers that all yielded LOD scores greater than 2.0, with the highest LOD occurring at *D16S749* (LOD=2.8). The authors note that this region is intriguing to investigators because there are several known candidate genes for bipolar disorder located here, including genes involved in neurotransmission. For example, two genes involved in γ-aminobutyric acid (GABA) transmission, which appears to be low in depressed and bipolar subjects (Berrettini et al. 1982, 1983, 1986), are located in this region.

Itokawa et al. (2003) examined a gene involved in *N*-methyl-D-aspartate subunit 1 receptor (NMDAR) expression, the GRIN2A promoter gene, located on 16p13.3. In this sample, association analysis of a panel of 96 multiplex bipolar pedigrees indicated a statistically significant bias in the transmission of longer alleles. The authors note that their results suggest that longer than average alleles result in hypoglutamatergic neurotransmission, which in turn contributes to bipolar susceptibility.

Also on 16p13, the adenylate cyclase type 9 gene (*ADCY9*) is a candidate gene for bipolar disorder because it is involved in neuronal signaling because it may be a target of antidepressants, and because mood stabilizers alter second messenger signals. However, findings from association studies have been ambiguous (Toyota et al. 2000, 2002b), and further investigation is needed to clarify whether this gene plays a role in bipolar disorder.

Chromosome 18

With regard to linkage studies, the most widely studied findings have been reported on chromosome 18. Berrettini and colleagues (1994) and Detera-Wadleigh et al. (1999) reported suggestive and significant linkage to the pericentromeric region of chromosome 18. Additionally, Costa Rican pedigrees supported linkage to the tip of 18p and 18q22–23 (Garner et al. 2001). The meta-analysis of Segurado et al. (2003) identified several regions on chromosome 18 as potentially encompassing susceptibility loci for bipolar disorder, including 18pter-p11 (under a narrow disease model, weighted and unweighted analyses) and 18p11–q12.3 (under all weighted models). Genes in this region potentially linked to bipolar disorder include *CHMP1.5* (Berrettini 2003) and *G-olf**, although several negative findings have been published regarding the role of *G-olf** in bipolar disorder (e.g., Turecki et al. 1996; Zill et al. 2003).

Chromosome 22

Several groups have reported suggestive to significant linkage to chromosome 22 in bipolar samples, including the NIMH Genetics Initiative samples, the NIMH neurogenetics pedigrees, and Kelsoe et al. (2001). In Badner and Gershon's (2002) meta-analysis of published whole-genome scans of bipolar disorder and schizophrenia, there was strong evidence for 22q harboring a common susceptibility locus for both disorders. Potash et al. (2003) also reported evidence of linkage in families with psychotic mood disorders to 22q12, reporting a nonparametric LOD score of 3.06; including families without psychotic mood disorders resulted in little evidence for linkage to this region. Badenhop et al. (2002) detected a two-point LOD of 2.0 on chromosome 22q11 at marker D22S420 under a recessive, broad model, but only within a single pedigree.

Several interesting candidate genes for bipolar disorder are located on chromosome 22. Lachman et al. (1996) found a relationship between an allele for a variant of the catechol *O*-methyltransferase (*COMT*) gene and rapid cycling in bipolar disorder (however, see also Biomed European Bipolar Collaborative Group 1997). In a study described previously, Rotondo et al. (2002) examined the frequency of the polymorphisms for the COMT gene in affected and unaffected groups. Relative to the healthy subjects, bipolar patients not comorbid for panic disorder had significantly higher frequencies of the COMT Met158 alleles. Recently, Barrett et al. (2003) examined the role of the G protein receptor kinase 3 gene (*GRK3*) in two independent sets of families with bipolar probands. An SNP was found to be associated with disease in the families of northern European descent in this sample.

Chromosome X

With a 1:1 equal gender distribution, it is counterintuitive to suggest that susceptibility for bipolar illness inheritance may be X-linked. However, there appears to an association whereby disease inherited from the father may be more severe, suggesting a possible contributing effect on the X chromosome.

Analyses of the NIMH Genetics Initiative pedigrees (waves 1 and 2; 153 families) support linkage to the X chromosome on Xp22.1, with a heterogeneity LOD of 2.3 (McInnis et al. 1999). More recently, Ekholm et al. (2002) conducted a further examination of the relationship between the X chromosome and bipolar disorder in a sample of Finnish families using a dense marker map. Subjects were 341 individuals from 41 bipolar families. Five diagnostic categories were used, reflecting increasingly broad inclusion criteria. Microsatellite markers were used, and parametric linkage analyses were conducted by using MLINK from the ANALYZE package (Hiekkalinna et al. 2005). Using a dominant model of inheritance, a suggestive maximum two-point LOD score of 2.78 was found at marker *DXS1047* under a model including bipolar I and schizoaffective disorders. Previous research from this group has also supported linkage between bipolar disorder and markers on Xq24–q27.1 (Pekkarinen et al. 1995). Zandi et al. (2003) reported a suggestive parametric heterogeneity LOD of 2.25 at marker *GATA144D04* under a narrow, recessive model.

Several association studies have examined candidate genes on the X chromosome. A dysfunction in GABA system activity has been hypothesized to play a role in bipolar vulnerability. Massat et al. (2002a) examined the GABA receptor (*GABRA3*) dinucleotide polymorphism, which maps to Xq28, in a matched European sample of 185 bipolar patients and 370 controls, and found that bipolar patients were much more likely to have one or more copies of allele 1 than control subjects.

THE REMAINDER OF THE GENOME

Chromosome 1

In 1999, Detera-Wadleigh et al. reported suggestive linkage to 1q31–32 in a genome-wide scan of 22 pedigrees. However, few recent studies have found linkage signals to chromosome 1 that meet standard criteria for significance (Lander and Kruglyak 1995). Ewald et al. (2002b) examined two families of bipolar probands of Danish Caucasian origin for genome-wide linkage using narrow and broad phenotypic models.

Two-point parametric analyses were conducted by using LINKAGE (Lathrop et al. 1984). Under a broad model, parametric analyses yielded a suggestive two-point LOD score of 2.75 for affected members only in both families at *D1S216,* and a follow-up three-point analysis detected an increased LOD score of 2.98. However, given that this sample consisted of only two families, these findings should be taken with caution.

In a genome-wide survey, Curtis et al. (2003) examined seven British and Icelandic pedigrees affected with multiple cases of bipolar disorder and unipolar depression, diagnosed by using the RDC (Spitzer et al. 1978). A total of 365 microsatellite markers were used, and VITESSE (O'Connell and Weeks 1995) was used for LOD score analyses. Bipolar depression, unipolar depression, and combined models were run assuming dominant or recessive transmission, for a total of 6 LOD score analyses. Results suggest a potential vulnerability locus in the region of marker *D1S251;* a four-point LOD score analysis revealed a suggestive peak heterogeneity LOD score of 2.0 under a combined, dominant model. The findings from both Ewald et al. (2002b) and Curtis et al. (2003) are consistent with earlier reports from the NIMH Genetics Initiative bipolar survey (Rice et al. 1997; Detera-Wadleigh et al. 1999).

Chromosome 2

Liu and colleagues (2003) examined a sample of 57 extended families (1,508 Caucasian individuals) with bipolar disorder in the United States and Israel. Diagnoses were made following the RDC. For their genome-wide screening, microsatellite markers were used, and two-point parametric analyses were carried out by using MLINK (Cottingham et al. 1993). They reported a suggestive LOD score of 3.20 for the region 2p13–16 using an intermediate disease phenotype and a dominant model of transmission. However, the multipoint LOD score for this region did not attain significance.

Chromosome 3

As part of an ongoing bipolar genetics study, Badenhop et al. (2002) analyzed a sample of 13 pedigrees comprised of 231 members. Families were Caucasian, generally of British or Irish descent, and diagnoses were made by using the RDC. Blood samples were genotyped using microsatellite markers. In a genome-wide linkage analysis by using ANALYZE (Hiekkalina et al. 2005), 3q25 showed evidence of linkage with a suggestive heterogeneity LOD score of 2.49 under a narrowly defined phenotype and an autosomal dominant inheritance model. These authors reported that this finding supports their previous reports of linkage findings in this region (Badenhop et al. 2001). Curtis et al. (2003) reported a suggestive peak heterogeneity LOD score of 2.0 around marker *D3S1265* for a combined, recessive model.

Chromosome 5

In an attempt to reproduce findings from earlier linkage analyses, Dick et al. (2002) analyzed a replication sample of 56 multiplex bipolar families from the NIMH Genetics Initiative for bipolar disorder. Microsatellite markers were used, and chromosomes 5, 15, 16, 17, and 22 were analyzed using nonparametric multipoint linkage analysis. Sibling-pair analysis by using ASPEX (Hinds and Risch 1999) revealed a suggestive LOD score of 2.8 for a broad disease model at marker *D5S207*. However, the LOD score for this marker decreased to 2.0 when the replication and original sample were combined for analysis of sibling-pairs with genotyped parents.

Greenwood et al. (2001) reported differential transmission of a marker of five SNPs within the dopamine transporter gene (*DAT*) on 5p15.3. More recently, because of its potential relevance to psychiatric disease, Ohtsuki and colleagues (2002) examined polymorphisms of the *HTR4* gene, which is on 5q32, in a case-control sample of 48 patients with mood disorder. Four polymorphisms at or in close proximity to exon *d* showed an association with bipolar disorder. However, some of these relationships were also present in patients with major depressive disorder, and the functional implications of these polymorphisms are unclear.

Chromosome 6

In an older study of an Amish pedigree, Ginns et al. (1996) reported suggestive linkage signals at marker *D6S7*. Another report of findings related to chromosome 6 comes from Dick et al. (2003), who conducted genome-wide linkage analyses on 1,152 individuals (mostly Caucasian) from 250 families in the multisite NIMH Genetics Initiative bipolar survey. Bipolar I disorder and SABP diagnostic criteria were derived from DSM-III-R, and bipolar II and recurrent major depression (UPR) were diagnosed following the RDC. Markers were adapted from the Cooperative Human Linkage Center marker set version 9, and nonparametric, multipoint linkage analysis using affected relative pairs was carried out by using Merlin (Abecasis et al. 2002). In this sample, chromosome 6 yielded a suggestive maximum LOD score of 2.2 (near marker *D6S1021*) under a broad disease model, using nonparametric, multipoint methods of linkage. A combined analysis of 399 NIMH pedigrees yields a significant LOD of 3.8 at 113cM on 6q (Hinrichs et al. unpublished data).

Chromosome 7

In the sample described earlier, Liu et al. (2003) ran affected sib-pair (ASP) analyses (by using MAPMAKER/SIBS; Kruglyak and Lander 1995) and reported a suggestive multipoint LOD score of 2.78 at 7q34 by using an intermediate disease phenotype. The authors noted that suggestive evidence for linkage to 7q has also been reported by Detera-Wadleigh et al. (1997; 1999).

Chromosome 8

In an effort to identify regions of linkage across multiple data sets, Segurado et al. (2003) applied meta-analytic techniques to 18 bipolar genome scans, including some unpublished studies. The authors used a ranking of binned areas within each genome scan to permit a nonparametric meta-analysis (for a more detailed description of the methods of this study, see Levinson et al. 2003). Studies were analyzed by using very narrow (bipolar I and SABP), narrow (adding bipolar II), and broad (adding UPR) models, in analyses weighted and unweighted for sample size. Although no chromosomal region attained genome-wide significance by simulation-based criteria, a region on chromosome 8q (8q24.21-qter) attained nominal significance under the narrow and broad models in the weighted analyses. Dick et al. (2003) reported a suggestive LOD score of 2.46 under a narrowly defined disease phenotype, near the marker *D8S256*. By using an intermediate model of disease, McInnis and colleagues (2003b) reported a suggestive nonparametric LOD of 2.1 on 8q24, also around the marker D8S256. Badenhop et al. (2002) reported a suggestive two-point heterogeneity LOD score of 2.08 around marker *D8S514* under a dominant, narrow model.

Chromosome 9

The Segurado et al. (2003) study described above produced weak findings for a region on chromosome 9p-q being linked to bipolar disorder. In weighted analyses, this region attained nominal statistical significance under a very narrow disease phenotype.

Lithium and valproate may produce some of their effects by action on NMDAR subunit 1; thus, genes that code for the subunits of the NM-DAR may be regarded as candidate genes for bipolar disorder. The NMDAR 1 subunit is coded by a gene on chromosome 9q34.3 (*GRIN1*). Mundo et al. (2003) examined three polymorphisms of this gene for linkage disequilibrium in bipolar disorder. A total of 288 probands with bipolar I or bipolar II disorder or schizoaffective disorder, manic type, and their parents were recruited from Canadian clinics. A preferential transmission of the G allele was found for the *1001G/C* and *6608G/C* variants of the *GRIN1* in affected individuals, suggesting these polymorphisms confer vulnerability to bipolar disorder. The authors note that these variants are silent substitutions and are unlikely to directly affect the NMDAR; thus, the functional implications of their findings are unclear.

Chromosome 10

McInnis et al. (2003a) conducted a genome-wide scan of 153 mostly Caucasian pedigrees as part of the NIMH Genetics Initiative for bipolar disorder. Markers were constructed by using CRIMAP (Lander and Green 1987), and GENEHUNTER-PLUS (Kong and Cox 1997) was used to compute nonparametric LOD scores. These investigators reported a suggestive LOD of 2.2 for the marker *D10S1423* on chromosome 10p12 under an intermediate disease model. This linkage was also reported by Foroud et al. (2000) in the first 97 pedigrees from the genetics initiative. This region of 10p has been implicated in linkage studies of schizophrenia as well (Faraone et al. 1998; Schwab et al. 1998).

Linkage to 10q has been reported by several groups, including Ewald et al. (1999) and Cichon et al. (2001). Using multipoint parametric analysis, Liu et al. (2003) obtained a suggestive LOD of 2.33 at 10q24 under a dominant, narrowly defined phenotype. However, a follow-up ASP analysis found a maximum LOD score of only 1.57 for this region. In their weighted meta-analysis, under a narrowly defined model, Segurado et al. (2003) found evidence that the region 10q11.21–q22.1 may contain genes with weak effects on bipolar disorder.

Toward clarifying the relationship between this region and bipolar disorder and schizophrenia, Ewald et al. (2002a) examined allelic association and chromosome segment and haplotype sharing on chromosome 10q26 in a sample of distantly related patients with schizophrenia or bipolar disorder and controls. In an isolated population sample on the Faroe Islands, patient lineages were traced back to determine familial relationships. Twenty-two microsatellite markers were used, and both assumption-free tests and tests based upon genealogical relationships were used. Allele frequency and haplotype segments were compared between patients and controls by using CLUMP (Sham and Curtis 1995). Comparing the combined patient group to the controls revealed an allelic association at marker *D10S1723*, which is consistent with the notion of a common susceptibility region for the two disorders. Another region between *D10S214* and *D10S505* showed evidence for increased haplotype sharing in bipolar disorder.

Chromosome 13

Evidence also exists to support linkage on chromosome 13. Stine and colleagues (1997) reported modest evidence of linkage to chromosome 13q32 in the NIMH Genetics Initiative pedigrees, and further support for this finding was reported by Detera-Wadleigh et al. (1999) in the Neurogenetics sample. Liu et al. (1999) and Kelsoe et al. (2001) have also reported suggestive findings of linkage on chromosome 13q.

With regard to more recent findings, in a sample of 65 probands with bipolar I disorder and 237 relatives affected with a major mood disorder, Potash et al. (2003) examined four chromosomal regions thought to confer genetic susceptibility to both schizophrenia and bipolar disorder. Diagnoses were made according to the RDC, and subsets of families were created based upon the number of members with psychotic mood disorder. Markers were microsatellite tandem repeats, and nonparametric linkage analysis was performed by using GENE-HUNTER (Kong and Cox 1997). The 10 families with three or more members with psychotic mood disorders showed suggestive evidence of linkage to 13q31, with a suggestive LOD score of 2.52, while these regions showed little evidence of linkage when the sample was examined in its entirety. Additionally, Badner and Gershon (2002) conducted a meta-analysis of published whole-genome scans of bipolar disorder and schizophrenia. The results show significant linkage for both disorders in the 13q region. Badenhop et al. (2002) reported a suggestive two-point LOD score of 2.29 for marker *D13S153* (on 13q14) under a recessive model with a broadly defined disease phenotype, and Liu et al. (2003) reported a suggestive multipoint ASP LOD score of 2.2 under an intermediate diagnostic model for the *D13S779* marker on 13q32.

Several association studies also implicate 13q in bipolar disorder. In an association study, Hattori et al. (2003) examined the relationship between the G72/G30 gene locus on 13q33 and bipolar disorder in two series of pedigrees, one from the Clinical Neurogenetics pedigrees (Berrettini et al. 1991), and another from the NIMH Genetic Initiative. The investigators performed transmission/disequilibrium testing

(TDT) and haplotype analysis. A similar haplotype was overtransmitted in both samples, which suggests that a susceptibility variant for bipolar disorder exists in this region. Given that several other papers have reported similar findings (Chen et al. 2004; Schumacher et al. 2004), it has recently been proposed that the relationship between the *G72/G30* complex and bipolar disorder be considered a conclusive finding (DePaulo 2004). Ranade et al. (2003) examined linkage and association between bipolar disorder and serotonin type 2A receptor gene polymorphisms in a sample of 93 patients from Pennsylvania clinics and their parents (either one or both). Comparing the bipolar patients to controls revealed an association with SNPs on exons 2 and 3, consistent with haplotype differences. Examining patients and their parents suggested significant linkage and association with *1354C/T* and haplotypes containing this SNP. These linkage and association studies suggest potential susceptibility loci somewhere on 13q, possibly for both bipolar disorder and schizophrenia or psychosis.

Chromosome 14

The Segurado et al. (2003) meta-analysis provided support for the hypothesis that a region on chromosome 14q may contain loci that modestly influence susceptibility to bipolar disorder. In their primary weighted analyses, the region 14q24.1–q32.12 attained nominal statistical significance under all the disease phenotypes examined in this study. However, no individual studies have reported significant linkage in this region.

Chromosome 15

Papadimitriou and colleagues (1998) reported an association with alleles of the GABA-A receptor alpha 5 subunit gene (*GABRA5*), which is on chromosome 15q11-q13, and bipolar disorder in a Greek sample of 48 bipolar patients and 50 control subjects.

In a sample of 31 bipolar patients who had an excellent response to lithium and their 247 relatives, Turecki et al. (2001) reported a significant LOD of 3.43 to 15q14 under a recessive model of inheritance.

Chromosome 17

Using multipoint, nonparametric linkage methods examining affected relative pairs, Dick et al. (2003) found suggestive evidence for linkage on chromosome 17q where they obtained a LOD score of 2.4 under an intermediate disease model. Liu et al. (2003) reported a two-point parametric LOD score of 2.68 at *D17S921* under a dominant model of narrowly defined disease. The multipoint LOD for this same locus and model increased slightly to 2.72.

In an earlier study, Collier et al. (1996) found an association of the short allele of the serotonin transporter (5-HTT) gene, which maps to 17q11.1–12, and bipolar and unipolar depression. Rotondo et al. (2002) examined *5HTT* in a sample of unrelated Italian bipolar patients with and without comorbid panic disorder ($n=49$ and $n=62$, respectively) and 127 healthy subjects. The frequency of the polymorphisms for *5HTT* were determined and compared between affected and unaffected groups. Relative to the healthy subjects, bipolar patients who were not comorbid for panic disorder had significantly higher frequencies of the short *5HTTLPR* alleles. This finding strengthens existing evidence for a role of *5HTT* polymorphisms in bipolar disorder, and suggests that "pure" bipolar disorder may represent a more homogenous phenotype with different genetic underpinnings than bipolar disorder comorbid with other conditions. Bellivier et al. (2002) also examined polymorphisms of the *5HTTLPR* in a sample of 223 bipolar, French, Caucasian patients classified as early, intermediate, or late age at onset. Patients homozygous for the short allele were found to have an earlier age of illness onset.

Chromosome 20

Willour et al. (2003) conducted further analysis of the 56 multiplex bipolar pedigrees from the wave 2 sample of the NIMH Genetics Initiative for bipolar disorder, examining chromosomes 4, 7, 9, 18, 19, 20, and 21. Nonparametric and parametric analyses were conducted with the program GENEHUNTER-PLUS (Kong and Cox 1997). While evidence for linkage was weak in the wave 2 sample alone, linkage analysis of the waves 1 and 2 samples combined detected a nonparametric LOD score of 2.38 at *D20S162*, under a broad disease model.

Chromosome 21

Straub et al. (1994) reported significant linkage to chromosome 21q22, and additional evidence for linkage to this region was observed by Detera-Wadleigh et al. (1996) in two independent samples. More recently, in an extension of the study of Straub et al. (1994), Liu and colleagues (2001) also reported evidence of linkage in 56 families to chromosome 21, finding a two-point LOD of 3.56 at *D21S1260*.

FUTURE DIRECTIONS

As can be concluded from the present review, numerous regions have at least some support as putative susceptibility loci in bipolar disorder, with 4, 11, 12q, 16, 18, 22q, and Xq arguably showing the most support. Studies have also provided evidence for numerous candidate genes playing a role in bipolar disorder, including the *G72/G30* complex, genes involved in the serotonergic and dopaminergic systems, *BDNF,* and *COMT* (see Table 3–1). However, while we have attempted to highlight recent significant findings of linkage and association, for many of the positive findings we report there are at least as many negative findings and replication failures. Given that risk for bipolar disorder is probably genetically heterogeneous, some variability in findings is to be expected; however, at least some of these findings will likely fail to receive further support in future studies. The question remains of how to conduct research in a way that minimizes misleading results while capturing the genuine complexity of the relationship between genes and bipolar disorder.

To date, no one approach has emerged as clearly superior in bipolar genetics research, and it is likely that a combination of study designs is required to elucidate the molecular bases for bipolar disorder. Thus, while we cannot endorse any one strategy over another, a preliminary step toward increasing the durability of findings in bipolar genetics studies is to use designs that accommodate the complexity and heterogeneity of bipolar disorder. For example, early studies of linkage in bipolar disorder used smaller samples of large families, as this relatively inexpensive approach had provided insight into illnesses following single-gene patterns of inheritance. As it seems clear now that the pattern of inheritance for bipolar disorder is inconsistent with a single gene, and that large families with bipolar disorder are probably not representative of families at risk for bipolar disorder, collaborative linkage studies have more recently concentrated on multiple, small families. Similarly, the practice of using population isolates, as opposed to more heterogeneous samples, was initially embraced as being more likely to lead to the identification of specific genes implicated in bipolar disorder. However, this strategy does not appear to have produced the expected results, and since such samples may be limited in their generalizability for larger bipolar populations, future studies may wish to de-emphasize this approach.

Also regarding the complexity of bipolar disorder, multiple theorists (e.g., Eysenck et al. 1983) have proposed that dimensional models of psychopathology may better capture the true nature of many psychiat-

TABLE 3–1. Overview of recent evidence for candidate genes for bipolar disorder

Gene	Location	Functional significance	Supportive evidence
DAT	5p	Mediates reuptake of dopamine	Greenwood et al. 2001
GRIN1	9q	*GRIN1* codes NMDAR1 subunit; lithium may act via NMDAR	Mundo et al. 2003
DRD4	11p	Dopamine system regulates emotion, motivation	Muglia et al. 2002
DRD2	11q	Same as above	Massat et al. 2002a
NCAM1	11q	*NCAM1* is involved in various neurodevelopmental processes; disruption of these may contribute to bipolar disorder	Arai et al. 2004
BDNF	11p	BDNF influences serotonergic system; involved in stress exposure, antidepressant response	Neves-Pereira et al. 2002; Sklar et al. 2002
G72/G30	13q	*G72* interacts with D-amino-acid oxidase; *G30* unknown	Chen et al. 2004; Hattori et al. 2003; Schumacher et al. 2004
HTR2A	13q	May mediate effects of serotonin reuptake inhibitors	Ranade et al. 2003
GABRA5	15q	GABAnergic neurons influence a host of other neurotransmitters that regulate mood	Papadimitriou et al. 1998
GRIN2A	16p	GRIN2A alleles affect glutamatergic neurotransmission	Itokawa et al. 2003
ADCY9	16p	Adenylate cyclases are involved in neuronal signaling; may be antidepressant targets	Toyota et al. 2002b
5HTT	17q	Alleles affect transcriptional efficiency of 5-HTT promoter	Bellivier et al. 2002; Collier et al. 1996; Rotondo et al. 2002
CHMP1.5	18p	Affects G-protein signaling	Berrettini 2003

TABLE 3–1. Overview of recent evidence for candidate genes for bipolar disorder *(continued)*

Gene	Location	Functional significance	Supportive evidence
COMT	22q	COMT alleles affect enzymatic activity	Lachman et al. 1996; Rotondo et al. 2002
GRK3	22q	GRK3 may regulate homeostatic brain response to dopamine	Barrett et al. 2003
GABRA3	Xq	Bipolar disorder may stem in part from GABA deficit	Massat et al. 2002b

Note. 5-HTT=serotonin transporter; BDNF=brain-derived neurotrophic factor; GABA=γ-aminobutyric acid; NCAM 1=neural cell adhesion molecule 1; NMDAR= N-methyl-D-aspartate subunit 1 receptor.

ric diseases, as well as being more informative and reliable. Even though bipolar disorder may be best conceptualized as a continuous construct, most studies examining the genetic bases for bipolar disorder treat it as a dichotomy. To be fair, this convention is consistent with all major diagnostic systems, and there is no consensus of how to go about creating a valid, dimensional bipolar disorder construct. However, studies of genes and bipolar disorder may benefit from increased use of methods that treat the phenotype as quantitative. Along these same lines, while it is widely acknowledged that risk for bipolar disorder likely results from the effects of multiple genes that interact with one another, few studies have examined multiple genes and their interaction effects. Methods that treat individual genetic effects as independent of one another are likely distorting the true relationship between gene loci and bipolar disorder, and such analyses may also lack sufficient power to detect effects. In particular, future association studies should likely de-emphasize the traditional approach of examining single genes in favor of studying multiple candidate genes and their interactive effects. Given that it may soon be feasible to conduct a genome-wide association study, this approach may potentially be put into practice sooner, rather than later.

A similar issue can be seen in the lack of studies examining both genetic and environmental influences on bipolar disorder. Although the influence of genes in bipolar disorder is clearly important, evidence has mounted suggesting that environmental factors also play a significant role. For example, expressed emotion has been shown to predict symptom changes in bipolar disorder (Miklowitz et al. 1988), and numerous studies have provided evidence that stressful life events predict bipolar episode onset (e.g., Amberlas 1979; Bebbington et al. 1993; Dunner et al. 1979). Additionally, Mortensen et al. (2003) recently reported an association between parental loss during childhood and bipolar disorder. Furthermore, evidence is also mounting to suggest that events not considered particularly stressful, and even positive events, may play a unique role in bipolar disorder. For example, Malkhoff-Schwartz et al. (1998) found an association between events that disrupted "social rhythms" (e.g., sleeping, eating) and onset of manic episodes, and Johnson et al. (2000) provided evidence suggesting that life events involving goal-attainment show a specific relationship to manic symptomatology. Despite these findings, and despite the fact that such gene-environment models are beginning to be successfully applied to unipolar depression (e.g., Caspi et al. 2003), very few studies have incorporated both environmental and genetic factors in predicting course and outcome of bipolar disorder. Including environmental factors may be especially enlightening when examining genes of small effect, which may achieve penetrance only when considered in conjunction with environmental factors. Sufficient research on psychosocial influences on bipolar disorder currently exists to suggest some useful starting points for multivariate studies.

Future studies of the genetics of bipolar disorder may benefit from using phenotypes of both increased specificity and increased breadth. For example, several studies have used the strategy of examining subgroups of bipolar patients based on factors such as early age of onset (Faraone et al. 2003), psychotic symptomatology (Potash et al. 2003), treatment response (Turecki et al. 2001), and comorbid anxiety disorders (Rotondo et al. 2002). Further exploration of these subtypes is needed to clarify whether narrowly defined phenotypes yield greater consistency of linkage and association findings.

Bipolar patients with comorbid alcohol abuse may be a particularly valuable phenotype for future study. This phenotype has received previous theoretical attention (e.g., Winokur et al. 1971), with empirical evidence accumulating to support the notion that this is an important subtype. Kendler et al. (1993a) reported a genetic correlation of 0.4–0.6 between major depression and alcoholism. Our analysis of the NIMH Genetics Initiative families has produced several intriguing findings about the nature of bipolar disorder and alcoholism comorbidity. In this data set, we have found that having a diagnosis of serious affective disorder increases risk for alcoholism, particularly in female probands (see Table 3-2), and that bipolar probands comorbid for alcoholism have an earlier age of onset. Relatives of probands with both bipolar disorder and alcoholism are at elevated risk for comorbid affective disorder and alcoholism, indicating that this pattern of comorbidity runs in families (see Table 3–3). Linkage analyses suggest that chromosomes 4 and 16 may contain loci that influence the comorbid phenotype, and we have previously reported linkage evidence on proximal chromosome 1 for an alcohol or depressive phenotype (Nurnberger et al. 2001). Conversely, noncomorbid families show evidence for linkage to chromosomes 10 and 17. We suspect that further use of this phenotype will provide additional evidence supporting the existence of unique genetic factors that contribute to comorbid bipolar disorder and alcoholism.

Expanding genetic studies of bipolar disorder to include endophenotypes (i.e., traits associated with the disease that are heritable, precede disease onset, and are present in unaffected relatives) may also prove to be a fruitful approach, because such traits may reflect the underlying genetic phenomena more closely than diagnostic criteria. In schizophrenia research, endophenotypes have received a great deal of attention but are less widely used in research on bipolar disorder. It is somewhat unclear at present which endophenotypes for bipolar disorder would prove most useful, but candidates include circadian rhythm disruption, response to sleep disruption and psychostimulants, tryptophan depletion, and white matter hyperintensities (Lenox et al. 2002; Gould and Manji 2003), as well as electroencephalographic asymmetries (Hayden et al. 2003), temperament (Johnson et al. 2000; Kwapil et al. 2000; Lozano and Johnson 2001), cortisol (Ellenbogen et al. 2004), and melatonin levels (Nurnberger et al. 1999).

SUMMARY

Bipolar disorder is a highly heritable condition, as demonstrated by twin, family, and adoption studies that consistently suggest a strong genetic component to the disorder. However, identification of the specific genetic mechanisms underlying bipolar disorder has proven elusive, with linkage and association findings often failing to replicate. Despite these inconsistencies, findings have emerged to suggest that several chromosomes contain susceptibility loci for bipolar disorder, notably 4, 11, 12q, 16, 18p, 18q, 22q, and Xq. Studies also provide evidence that the *G72/G30* complex, *BDNF, GRK3,* and several genes involved in serotonin and dopamine neurotransmission are plausible candidate genes. Increased use of research designs that capture the complexity of bipolar disorder is recommended, such as studies examining gene-gene and gene-environment interactions. The use of phenotypes of greater speci-

TABLE 3–2. Comorbid alcoholism and affective disorder in the National Institute of Mental Health genetics bipolar data set

Affective diagnosis	DSM-III-R alcohol dependence, % (n)		Relative risk (95% confidence interval)	
	Males (n=3,411)	Females (n=3,929)	Males	Females
SABP	30.9 (21/68)	27.4 (20/73)	2.1 (1.3–3.5)*	10.1 (5.5–18.3)**
BPI	38.6 (307/796)	24.3 (294/1211)	2.8 (2.3–3.3)**	9.1 (6.3–13.1)**
BPII	37.4 (40/107)	22.8 (48/211)	3.0 (2.2–4.0)**	8.5 (5.4–13.4)**
UPR	31.7 (51/161)	14.3 (52/363)	2.5 (1.9–3.4)**	5.9 (3.7–9.3)**
UPS	35.0 (34/97)	5.0 (8/160)	2.4 (1.8–3.3)**	1.8 (0.8–3.8)
All major affective disorders	37.0 (453/1,229)	20.9 (422/2,018)	2.7 (2.3–3.1)**	7.1 (5.0–10.1)**
No major affective disorder	12.2 (266/2,182)	2.9 (55/1,911)	—	—

Note. BPI=bipolar I disorder; BPII=bipolar II disorder; SABP=schizoaffective disorder, bipolar subtype; UPR=recurrent unipolar depression; UPS=single episode, unipolar depression.
*P<0.01. **P<0.0001.

TABLE 3–3. Comorbidity in the relatives of bipolar probands comorbid and not comorbid for alcohol dependence

Bipolar probands	Probands' relatives with AD and major affective disorder, % (n)	Relative risk (95% confidence interval)
Comorbid AD	10.3 (211/2,049)	1.3 (1.1–1.6)*
Without comorbid AD	7.8 (330/4,218)	—

Note. Major affective disorder includes schizoaffective disorder (bipolar subtype), bipolar I disorder, bipolar II disorder, or recurrent unipolar depression. AD=DSM-III-R alcohol dependence.
*χ^2 (1)=10.7, $P<0.001$.

ficity, such as bipolar disorder with comorbid alcohol dependence, is recommended, as is the examination of endophenotypes.

REFERENCES

Abecasis GR, Cherny SS, Cookson WO, et al: Merlin-rapid analysis of dense genetic maps using sparse gene flow trees. Nat Genet 30:97–101, 2002

Adams LJ, Mitchell PB, Fielder SL, et al: A susceptibility locus for bipolar affective disorder on chromosome 4q35. Am J Hum Genet 62:1084–1091, 1998

Amberlas A: Psychologically stressful events in the precipitation of manic episodes. Br J Psychiatry 135:15–21, 1979

Arai M, Itokawa M, Yamada K, et al: Association of neural cell adhesion molecule 1 gene polymorphisms with bipolar affective disorder in Japanese individuals. Biol Psychiatry 55:804–810, 2004

Badenhop RF, Moses MJ, Scimone A, et al: A genome screen of a large bipolar affective disorder pedigree supports evidence for a susceptibility locus on chromosome 13q. Mol Psychiatry 6:396–403, 2001

Badenhop RF, Moses MJ, Scimone A, et al: A genome screen of 13 bipolar affective disorder pedigrees provides evidence for susceptibility loci on chromosome 3 as well as chromosomes 9, 13 and 19. Mol Psychiatry 7:851–859, 2002

Badenhop RF, Moses MJ, Scimone A, et al: Genetic refinement and physical mapping of a 2.3 Mb probable disease region associated with a bipolar affective disorder susceptibility locus on chromosome 4q35. Am J Med Genet 117:23–32, 2003

Badner JA, Gershon ES: Meta-analysis of whole genome linkage scans of bipolar disorder and schizophrenia. Mol Psychiatry 7:405–411, 2002

Barden N: Functional genomics of bipolar disorder. Am J Med Genet B Neuropsychiatr Genet 122:6, 2003

Barrett TB, Hauger RL, Kennedy JL, et al: Evidence that a single nucleotide polymorphism in the promoter of the G protein receptor kinase 3 gene is associated with bipolar disorder. Mol Psychiatry 8:546–557, 2003

Bebbington P, Wilkins S, Jones P: Life events and psychosis: Initial results from the Camberwell Collaborative Psychosis Study. Br J Psychiatry 162:72–79, 1993

Bellivier F, Leroux M, Henry C, et al: Serotonin transporter gene polymorphism influences age at onset in patients with bipolar affective disorder. Neurosci Lett 334:17–20, 2002

Berrettini WH: Chromosome 18p11 in bipolar disorder and schizophrenia. Am J Med Genet 122:6, 2003

Berrettini WH, Nurnberger JI Jr, Hare TA, et al: Plasma and CSF GABA in affective illness. Br J Psychiatry 141:483–487, 1982

Berrettini WH, Nurnberger JI Jr, Hare TA, et al: Reduced plasma and CSF GABA in affective illness: effect of lithium carbonate. Biol Psychiatry 18:185–194, 1983

Berrettini WH, Nurnberger JI Jr, Hare TA, et al: CSF GABA in euthymic manic-depressive patients and controls. Biol Psychiatry 21:844–846, 1986

Berrettini WH, Golden LR, Martinez MM, et al: A bipolar pedigree series for genomic mapping of disease genes: diagnostic and analytic considerations. Psychiatr Genet 2:125–160, 1991

Berrettini WH, Ferraro TN, Goldin LR, et al: Chromosome 18 DNA markers and manic depressive illness: evidence for a susceptibility gene. Proc Natl Acad Sci U S A 91:5918–5921, 1994

Bertelsen A, Harvald B, Hauge M: A Danish twin study of manic-depressive disorders. Br J Psychiatry 130:330–351, 1977

Biomed European Bipolar Collaborative Group: No association between bipolar disorder and alleles at a functional polymorphism in the COMT gene. Br J Psychiatry 170:526–528, 1997

Blackwood DH, He L, Morris SW, et al: A locus for bipolar disorder on chromosome 4p. Nat Genet 12:427–430, 1996

Cardno AG, Marshall EJ, Coid B, et al: Heritability estimates for psychotic disorders. Arch Gen Psychiatry 56:162–168, 1999

Caspi A, Sugden K, Moffitt TE, et al: Influence of life stress on depression: Moderation by a polymorphism in the 5-HTT gene. Science 301:386–389, 2003

Chen YS, Akula N, Detera-Wadleigh SD, et al: Findings in an independent sample support an association between bipolar affective disorder and the G72/G30 locus on chromosome 13q33. Mol Psychiatry 9:87–92, 2004

Cichon S, Schumacher J, Muller DJ, et al: A genome screen for genes predisposing to bipolar affective disorder detects a new susceptibility locus on 8q. Hum Mol Genet 10:2933–2944, 2001

Collier DA, Stober G, Heils A, et al: A novel functional polymorphism within the promoter of the serotonin transporter gene: possible role in susceptibility to affective disorders. Mol Psychiatry 1:453–460, 1996

Cottingham RW, Idury RM, Schaffer AA: Faster sequential genetic linkage computations. Am J Hum Genet 53:252–263, 1993

Craddock N, Jacobsen N, Franks E, et al: Molecular genetic investigation of bipolar disorder in the region of the Darier's disease gene (ATP2A2) on chromosome 12q23-q24.1. Mol Psychiatry 4:S71, 1999

Curtis D, Kalsi G, Brynjolfsson J, et al: Genome scan of pedigrees multiply affected with bipolar disorder provides further support for the presence of a susceptibility locus on chromosome 12q23-q24, and suggests the presence of additional loci on 1p and 1q. Psychiatr Genet 13:77–84, 2003

DePaulo JR: Genetics of bipolar disorder: where do we stand? Am J Psychiatry 161:595–597, 2004

Detera-Wadleigh S, Badner JA, Goldin LR, et al: Affected sib-pair analyses reveal support of prior evidence for susceptibility locus for bipolar disorder on 21q. Am J Hum Genet 58:1279–1285, 1996

Detera-Wadleigh SD, Badner JA, Yoshikawa T, et al: Initial genome scan of the NIMH Genetics Initiative bipolar pedigrees: Chromosomes 4, 7, 9, 18, 19, 20, and 21q. Am J Med Genet 74:254–262, 1997

Detera-Wadleigh SD, Badner JA, Berrettini WH, et al: A high-density genome scan detects evidence for a bipolar disorder susceptibility locus on 13q32 and other potential loci on 1q32 and 18p11.2. Proc Natl Acad Sci USA 96:5604–5609, 1999

Dick DM, Foroud T, Edenberg HJ, et al: Apparent replication of suggestive linkage on chromosome 16 in the NIMH Genetics Initiative bipolar pedigrees. Am J Med Genet 114:407–412, 2002

Dick DM, Foroud T, Flury L, et al: Genomewide linkage analyses of bipolar disorder: a new sample of 250 pedigrees from the National Institute of Mental Health Genetics Initiative. Am J Hum Genet 73:107–114, 2003

Dunner DL, Patrick V, Fieve RR: Life events at the onset of bipolar affective disorder. Am J Psychiatry 136:508–511, 1979

Einat H, Yuan P, Gould TD, et al: The role of the extracellular signal-regulated kinase signaling pathway in mood modulation. J Neurosci 23:7311–7316, 2003

Ekholm JM, Pekkarinen P, Pajukanta P, et al: Bipolar disorder susceptibility region on Xq24-q27.1 in Finnish families. Mol Psychiatry 7:453–459, 2002

Ellenbogen MA, Hodgins S, Walker C-D: High levels of cortisol among adolescent offspring of parents with bipolar disorder: a pilot study. Psychoneuroendocrinology 29:99–106, 2004

Ewald H, Flint T, Degn B, et al: A search for a shared segment of a chromosome 10q in patients with bipolar affective disorder from the Faroe Islands. Mol Psychiatry 4:S72, 1999

Ewald H, Flint TJ, Jorgensen TH, et al: Search for a shared segment on chromosome 10q26 in patients with bipolar affective disorder or schizophrenia from the Faroe Islands. Am J Med Genet 114:196–204, 2002a

Ewald H, Flint T, Kruse TA, et al: A genome-wide scan shows significant linkage between bipolar disorder and chromosome 12q24.3 and suggestive linkage to chromosomes 1p22–21, 4p16, 6q14–22, 10q26 and 16p13.3. Mol Psychiatry 7:734–744, 2002b

Eysenck HJ, Wakefield JA, Friedman AF: Diagnosis and clinical assessment: the DSM-III. Annu Rev Psychol 34:167–193, 1983

Faraone SV, Matise T, Svrakic D, et al: Genome scan of European American schizophrenia pedigrees: results of the NIMH Genetics Initiative and Millennium Consortium. Am J Med Genet 81:290–295, 1998

Faraone SV, Glatt SJ, Tsuang MT: The genetics of pediatric-onset bipolar disorder. Biol Psychiatry 53:970–977, 2003

Foroud T, Castelluccio PF, Koller DL, et al: Suggestive evidence of a locus on chromosome 10p using the NIMH Genetics Initiative bipolar affective disorder pedigrees. Am J Med Genet 96:18–23, 2000

Garner C, McInnes LA, Service SK, et al: Linkage analysis of a complex pedigree with severe bipolar disorder, using a Markov Chain Monte Carlo method. Am J Hum Genet 68:1061–1064, 2001

Gershon ES, Berrettini W, Nurnberger JI Jr, et al: Genetics of affective illness, in Psychopharmocology: The Third Generation of Progress. Edited by Meltzer HY. New York, Raven, 1987, pp 481–491

Ginns EI, Ott J, Egeland JA, et al: A genome-wide search for chromosomal loci linked to bipolar affective disorder in the Old Order Amish. Nat Genet 12:431–435, 1996

Gizatullin R, Zaboli G, Jonsson EG, et al: Haplotype analysis reveals tryptophan hydroxylase (TPH) 1 gene variants associated with major depression. Biol Psychiatry S9:295–300, 2006

Gould TD, Manji HK: The current status of endophenotypes in bipolar disorder. Am J Med Genet 122B:11, 2003

Greenwood TA, Alexander M, Keck PE, et al: Evidence for linkage disequilibrium between the dopamine transporter and bipolar disorder. Am J Med Genet 105:145–151, 2001

Hattori E, Liu C, Badner JA, et al: Polymorphisms at the G72/G30 locus, on 13q33, are associated with bipolar disorder in two independent pedigree series. Am J Hum Genet 72:1131–1140, 2003

Hayden EP, Hetrick WP, O'Donnell BF, et al: An examination of the convergent validity of questionnaire measures, behavioral tasks, and EEG indices of the behavioral activation system in a sample of patients with bipolar disorder. Poster presented at the 18th annual meeting of the Society for Research in Psychopathology, Toronto, ON, Canada, October 2003

Hiekkalinna T, Terwilliger JD, Sammalito S, et al: AUTOGSCAN: powerful tools for automated genome-wide linkage and linkage disequilibrium analysis. Twin Res Hum Genet 8:16–21, 2005

Hinds D, Risch N: The ASPEX package: affected sib-pair exclusion mapping. Available at http://aspex.sourceforge.net/. Accessed March 2006.

Itokawa M, Yamada K, Iwayama-Shigeno Y, et al: Genetic analysis of a functional GRIN2A promoter (GT)n repeat in bipolar disorder pedigrees in humans. Neurosci Lett 345:53–56, 2003

Jacobsen NJO, Franks EKE, Jones I, et al: Exclusion of the Darier's disease gene, ATP2A2, as a common susceptibility gene for bipolar disorder. Mol Psychiatry 6:92–97, 2001

Johnson SL, Sandrow D, Meyer B, et al: Increases in manic symptoms after life events involving goal attainment. J Abnorm Psychol 109:721–727, 2000

Jones J, Jacobsen N, Green EK, et al: Evidence for familial cosegregation of major affective disorder and genetic markers flanking the gene for Darier's disease. Mol Psychiatry 7:424–427, 2002

Kato T, Iwamoto K, Washizuka S, et al: No association of mutations and mRNA expression of WFS1/wolframin with bipolar disorder in humans. Neuroscience Lett 338:21–24, 2003

Keller MB, Lavori PW, Kane JM, et al: Subsyndromal symptoms in bipolar disorder. Arch Gen Psychiatry 49:371–376, 1992

Kelsoe JR, Spence MA, Loetscher E, et al: A genome survey indicates a possible susceptibility locus for bipolar disorder on chromosome 22. Proc Natl Acad Sci U S A 98:585–590, 2001

Kendler KS, Heath AC, Neale MC, et al: Alcoholism and major depression in women: a twin study of the causes of comorbidity. Arch Gen Psychiatry 50:690–698, 1993a

Kendler KS, Neale M, Kessler R, et al: A twin study of recent life events and difficulties. Arch Gen Psychiatry 50:789–796, 1993b

Kong A, Cox NJ: Allele-sharing models: LOD scores and accurate linkage tests. Am J Hum Genet 61:1179–1188, 1997

Kruglyak L, Lander ES: Complete multipoint sib-pair analysis of qualitative and quantitative traits. Am J Hum Genet 57:439–454, 1995

Kwapil TR, Miller MB, Zinser MC, et al: A longitudinal study of high scorers on the hypomanic personality scale. J Abnorm Psychol 109:222–226, 2000

Lachman HM, Morrow B, Shprintzen R, et al: Association of codon 108/158 catechol-O-methyltransferase gene polymorphism with the psychiatric manifestations of velo-cardio-facial syndrome. Am J Med Genet 67:468–472, 1996

Lai T-J, Wu C-Y, Tsai H-W, et al. Polymorphism screening and haplotype analysis of the tryptophan hydroxylase gene (TPH1) and association with bipolar affective disorder in Taiwan. BMC Medical Genetics 6:14, 2005

Lander ES, Green P: Construction of multilocus genetic linkage maps in humans. Proc Natl Acad Sci 84:2363–2367, 1987

Lander E, Kruglyak L: Genetic dissection of complex traits: guidelines for interpreting and reporting linkage results. Nat Genet 11:241–247, 1995

Lathrop GM, Lalouel JM, Julier C, et al: Strategies for multilocus linkage analysis in humans. Proc Natl Acad Sci 81:3443–3446, 1984

Lenox RH, Gould TD, Manji HK: Endophenotypes in bipolar disorder. Am J Med Genet 114:391–406, 2002; erratum Am J Med Genet 114:592, 2002

Levinson DF, Levinson MD, Seguardo R, et al: Genome scan meta-analysis of schizophrenia and bipolar disorder, I: methods and power analysis. Am J Hum Genet 73:17–33, 2003

Liu J, Aita VM, Knowles JA, et al: Search for susceptibility loci in extended pedigrees with bipolar affective disorder. Mol Psychiatry 4:S21, 1999

Liu J, Juo SH, Terwilliger JD, et al: A follow-up linkage study supports evidence for a bipolar affective disorder locus on chromosome 21q22. Am J Med Genet 105:189–194, 2001

Liu J, Juo SH, Dewan A, et al: Evidence for a putative bipolar disorder locus on 2p13–16 and other potential loci on 4q31, 7q34, 8q13, 9q31, 10q21–24, 13q32, 14q21 and 17q11–12. Mol Psychiatry 8:333–342, 2003

Lozano BE, Johnson SL: Can personality traits predict increases in manic and depressive symptoms? J Affect Disord 63:103–111, 2001

Malkhoff-Schwartz S, Frank E, Anderson B, et al: Stressful life events and social rhythm disruption in the onset of manic and depressive bipolar episodes: a preliminary investigation. Arch Gen Psychiatry 55: 702–707, 1998

Massat I, Souery D, Del-Favero J, et al: Excess of allele 1 for α_3 subunit GABA receptor gene (GABRA3) in bipolar patients: a multicentric association study. Mol Psychiatry 7:201–207, 2002a

Massat I, Souery D, Del-Favero J, et al: Positive association of dopamine D2 receptor polymorphism with bipolar affective disorder in a European multicenter association study of affective disorders. Am J Med Genet 114:177–185, 2002b

McInnis MG, MacKinnon DF, McMahon FJ, et al: Evidence for a susceptibility loci for bipolar disorder on the X chromosome. Mol Psychiatry 4:S75, 1999

McInnis M, Dick DM, Willour VL, et al: Genome-wide scan and conditional analysis in bipolar disorder: evidence for genomic interaction in the National Institute of Mental Health Genetics Initiative bipolar pedigrees. Biol Psychiatry 54:1265–1273, 2003a

McInnis M, Lan T-H, Willour VL, et al: Genome-wide scan of bipolar disorder in 65 pedigrees: supportive evidence for linkage at 8q24, 18q22, 4q32, 2p12, and 13q12. Mol Psychiatry 8:288–298, 2003b

Meloni R, Leboyer M, Bellivier F, et al: Association of manic-depressive illness with tyrosine hydroxylase microsatellite marker. Lancet 345:932, 1995

Mendelwicz J, Rainer JD: Adoption study supporting genetic transmission in manic-depressive illness. Nature 368:327–329, 1977

Miklowitz DJ, Goldstein MJ, Nuechterlien KH, et al: Family factors and the course of bipolar affective disorder. Arch Gen Psychiatry 45: 225–231, 1988

Morissette J, Villeneuve A, Bordeleau L, et al: Genome-wide search for linkage of bipolar affective disorders in a very large pedigree derived from a homogeneous population in Quebec points to a locus of major effect on chromosome 12q23-q24. Am J Med Genet 88:567–587, 1999

Mortensen PB, Pedersen CB, Melbye M, et al: Individual and familial risk factors for bipolar affective disorders in Denmark. Arch Gen Psychiatry 60:1209–1215, 2003

Muglia P, Petronis A, Mundo E, et al: Dopamine D4 receptor and tyrosine hydroylase genes in bipolar disorder: evidence for a role of DRD4. Mol Psychiatry 7:860–866, 2002

Mundo E, Tharmalingham S, Neves-Pereira M, et al: Evidence that the N-methyl-D-aspartate subunit 1 receptor gene (GRIN1) confers susceptibility to bipolar disorder. Mol Psychiatry 8:241–245, 2003

Murray CJL, Lopez AD (eds): The Global Burden of Disease: A Comprehensive Assessment of Mortality and Disability From Diseases, Injuries, and Risk Factors in 1990 and Projected to 2020. Boston, MA, Harvard University Press, 1996

Nakata K, Ujike H, Sakai A, et al: Association study of the brain-derived neurotrophic factor (BDNF) gene with bipolar disorder. Neurosci Lett 337:17–20, 2003

Nanko S, Yokoyama H, Hoshino Y, et al: Organic mood syndrome in two siblings with Wolfram syndrome. Br J Psychiatry 161:282, 1992

Neves-Pereira M, Mundo E, Muglia P, et al: The brain-derived neurotrophic factor gene confers susceptibility to bipolar disorder: evidence from a family based association study. Am J Hum Genet 71:651–655, 2002

Nurnberger JI Jr, Adkins S, Lahiri DK, et al: Melatonin suppression by light in euthymic bipolar and unipolar patients. Arch Gen Psychiatry 57:572–579, 2000

Nurnberger JI Jr, Foroud T, Flury L, et al: Evidence for a locus on chromosome 1 that influences vulnerability to alcoholism and affective disorder. Am J Psychiatry 158:718–724, 2001

O'Connell JR, Weeks DE: The VITESSE algorithm for rapid exact multilocus linkage analysis via genotype set-recoding and fuzzy inheritance. Nat Genet 11:402–408, 1995

Ohtsuki T, Ishiguro H, Detera-Wadleigh SD, et al: Association between serotonin 4 receptor gene polymorphisms and bipolar disorder in Japanese case-control samples and the NIMH genetics initiative bipolar pedigrees. Mol Psychiatry 7:954–961, 2002

Papadimitriou GN, Dikeos DG, Karadima G, et al. Association between the GABA-A receptor α_5 subunit gene locus (GABRA5) and bipolar affective disorder. Am J Med Genet 81:73–80, 1998

Pekkarinen P, Terwilliger J, Bredbacka PE, et al: Evidence of a predisposing locus to bipolar disorder on Xq24-q27.1 in an extended Finnish pedigree. Genome Res 5:105–115, 1995

Poltorak M, Khoja I, Hemperly JJ, et al: Disturbances in cell recognition molecules (N-CAM and L1 antigen) in the CSF of patients with schizophrenia. Exp Neurol 131:266–272, 1995

Potash JB, Zandi PP, Willour VL, et al: Suggestive linkage to chromosomal regions 13q31 and 22q12 in families with psychotic bipolar disorder. Am J Psychiatry 160:680–686, 2003

Ranade SS, Mansour H, Wood J, et al: Linkage and association between serotonin 2A receptor gene polymorphisms and bipolar I disorder. Am J Med Genet 121:28–34, 2003

Rice JP, Goate A, Williams JT, et al: Initial genome scan of the NIMH Genetics Initiative bipolar pedigrees: chromosomes 1, 6, 8, 10, and 12. Am J Med Genet 74:247–253, 1997

Rotondo A, Mazzanti C, Dell'Osso L, et al: Catechol O-methyltransferase, serotonin transporter, and tryptophan hydroxylase gene polymorphisms in bipolar disorder patients with and without comorbid panic disorder. Am J Psychiatry 159:23–29, 2002

Schumacher J, Abon Jamra R, Freudenberg J, et al: Examination of G72 and D-amino-acid oxidase as genetic risk factors for schizophrenia and bipolar affective disorder. Mol Psychiatry 9:203–207, 2004

Schwab SG, Hallmayer J, Albus M, et al: Further evidence for a susceptibility locus on chromosome 10p14-p11 in 72 families with schizophrenia by nonparametric linkage analysis. Am J Med Genet 81:302–307, 1998

Segurado R, Detera-Wadleigh SD, Levinson DF, et al: Genome scan meta-analysis of schizophrenia and bipolar disorder, III: bipolar disorder. Am J Hum Genet 73:49–62, 2003

Sham PC, Curtis D: An extended transmission/disequilibrium test (TDT) for multi-allele marker loci. Ann Hum Genet 59:97–105, 1995

Sklar P, Gabriel SB, McInnis MG, et al: Family based association study of 76 candidate genes in bipolar disorder: BDNF is a potential risk locus. Mol Psychiatry 7:579–593, 2002

Spitzer R, Endicott J, Robins E: Research diagnostic criteria: rationale and reliability. Arch Gen Psychiatry 35:773–782, 1978

Stine OC, McMahon FJ, Chen L, et al: Initial genome screen for bipolar disorder in the NIMH Genetics Initiative pedigrees: chromosomes 2, 11, 13, 14, and X. Am J Med Genet 74:263–269, 1997

Straub RE, Lehner T, Luo Y, et al: A possible vulnerability locus for bipolar affective disorder on chromosome 21q22.3. Nat Genet 8:291–296, 1994

Toyota T, Watanabe A, Shibuya H, et al: Association study on the DUSP6 gene, an affective disorder candidate gene on 12q23, performed by using flouresence resosnance energy transfer-based melting curve analysis on the LightCycler. Mol Psychiatry 5:489–494, 2000

Toyota T, Hattori E, Meerabux J, et al: Molecular analysis, mutation screening, and association study of adenylate cyclase type 9 gene (ADCY9) in mood disorders. Am J Med Genet 114:84–92, 2002a

Toyota T, Yamada K, Saito K, et al: Association analysis of adenylate cyclase type 9 gene using pedigree disequilibrium test in bipolar disorder. Mol Psychiatry 7:450–452, 2002b

Turecki G, Alda M, Grof P, et al: No association between chromosome-18 markers and lithium-responsive affective disorders. Psychiatry Res 63:17–23, 1996

Turecki G, Grof P, Grof E, et al: Mapping susceptibility genes for bipolar disorder: a pharmacogenetic approach based on excellent response to lithium. Mol Psychiatry 6:570–578, 2001

Wender PH, Kety SS, Rosenthal D, et al: Psychiatric disorders in the biological and adoptive families of adopted individuals with affective disorders. Arch Gen Psychiatry 43:923–929, 1986

Willour VL, Zandi PP, Huo Y, et al: Genome scan of the fifty-six bipolar pedigrees from the NIMH Genetics Initiative replication sample: Chromosomes 4, 7, 9, 18, 20, and 21. Am J Med Genet 121:21–27, 2003

Willner P, Muscat R, Phillips G: The role of dopamine in rewarded behavior: ability, insight, drive or incentive? Pol J Pharmacol Pharm 43:291–300, 1991

Willner P, Muscat R, Papp M: An animal model of anhedonia. Clin Neuropharmacol 15a:550–551, 1992

Winokur G, Cadoret R, Dorzab J, et al: Depressive disease: a genetic study. Arch Gen Psychiatry 24:135–144, 1971

Wyatt RJ, Henter I: An economic evaluation of manic-depressive illness: 1991. Social Psychiatry Psychiatr Epidemiol 30:213–219, 1995

Zandi PP, Willour VL, Huo Y, et al: Genome scan of a second wave of NIMH Genetics Initiative bipolar pedigrees: chromosomes 2, 11, 13, 14, and X. Am J Med Genet 119:69–76, 2003

Zill P, Malitas PN, Bondy B, et al: Analysis of polymorphisms in the alpha-subunit of the olfactory G-protein Golf in lithium-treated bipolar patients. Psychiatric Genet 13:65–69, 2003

SPECIAL TOPICS IN BIPOLAR DEPRESSION

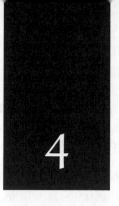

4

PEDIATRIC BIPOLAR DEPRESSION

Anoop Karippot, M.D.

ALTHOUGH AFFECTIVE DISORDERS IN youths are lately receiving much more attention, they continue to be a diagnostic puzzle. It is estimated that 5% of children and adolescents suffer from major depression, 4% from dysthymia, and 1% from bipolar depression (Lewinsohn et al. 1993). Depression in children and adolescents is a serious condition, associated with considerable morbidity and mortality (Kovacs 1996). As discussed in Chapter 1, "Diagnosis of Bipolar Depression," bipolar depression as a clinical entity is underdiagnosed in adults and commonly undiagnosed in children.

Pediatric depression was not officially recognized until 1975 (Raskin et al. 1978). Since then, it has been conclusively documented both in the psychiatric community and in clinical settings (Angold 1988a, 1988b; Fleming and Offord 1990). The decision to utilize adult criteria to diagnose depression in children can be traced to a 1975 conference at the National Institute of Mental Health, and the practice continues in DSM-IV-TR, in which the same diagnostic criteria for major depression applies both to children and adults. However, depending on the level of their maturity, language skills, and social skills, children tend to express depressive symptoms differently from adults.

Depressive episodes are the most common manifestation of bipolar affective disorders in children and adults alike. Distinguishing the differences between unipolar and bipolar forms of depression in children is a challenge. Bipolar depression is often undiagnosed or misdiagnosed as unipolar depression in both adults and children, resulting in incorrect or inadequate treatment—for example, the use of antidepressants to treat symptoms of depression in bipolar youths may actually precipitate mania (Biederman et al. 2000; Geller et al. 1994, 2001a; Strober et al. 1993). This illustrates the clinical relevance of correctly diagnosing pediatric bipolar depression.

Some studies have suggested that major depression with early childhood onset is associated with the subsequent development of bipolar disorder. In a prospective longitudinal study of 60 hospitalized, depressed adolescents aged 13–16 years, Strober et al. (1993) found that 20% of patients were rediagnosed with bipolar disorder at 3- to 4-year follow-up. The authors noted that the switch of diagnosis was predicted by the rapid onset of depressive symptoms, psychomotor retardation, mood-congruent psychotic features, a family history of bipolar illness, and a history of pharmacologically induced hypomania.

A similar finding was reported by Geller et al. (1994, 2001b): they followed 79 children (80% were prepubertal) with major depression and found that 32% switched to mania by an average age of 11 years and 50% by the age of 21 years. The predictors of diagnostic conversion in this study were conduct disorder, bullying, and a family history of bipolar disorder. Luby and Mrakotsky (2003) studied a group of depressed preschoolers and suggested that increased rates of restlessness seen in the depressed preschoolers with a family history of bipolar disorder may actually be a precursor of bipolar disorder.

These studies suggest that pediatric depressive symptoms, especially for children with a family history of bipolar disorder, are strongly associated with the later development of mania. The diagnosis of depression at an early age in childhood appears to indicate poor prognosis.

EPIDEMIOLOGY

Child and adolescent bipolar disorder have been less studied than adult-onset bipolar illness (Sanchez 1999). In adults, the prevalence of bipolar type I disorder is considered to be approximately 1% of the population; the rate of the illness in children is a matter of debate. Some studies indicate rates as high as 3.0%–6.5% for the bipolar spectrum (Hirschfeld et al. 2003).

Lewinsohn et al. (1995) conducted a large-scale, epidemiological study of bipolar disorder in adolescents. The lifetime prevalence of bipolar disorders in this study was approximately 1%, which was similar to that reported in the Epidemiologic Catchment Area Study (Weissman et al. 1988). Lewinsohn et al. (1995) studied 1,709 youths. Eighteen bipolar cases were detected (age 14–18 years) and the mean age of onset was 12±3 years. Only two subjects (11%) met the criteria for bipolar I disorder. More than half of these patients received mental health care, but only one was treated with lithium. The ratio of first-episode depressive patients versus manic patients was 61% to 5%. The bipolar patients had increased rates of comorbid separation anxiety and panic and disruptive behavior (especially attention-deficit/hyperactivity) disorders. The bipolar patients reported a significantly earlier age at onset of any psychiatric symptom, and about 44% had attempted suicide and had a more severe course.

The peak age at onset of bipolar disorder is believed to be between 15 and 19 years. Lish et al. (1994) surveyed 500 members of a national depressive association who had bipolar disorder and the peak age at onset of bipolar disorder symptoms was indeed in the teenage years. A family history of bipolar disorder predicted early onset of depressive (33%) or mixed symptoms and was associated with a difficult course of illness in adulthood. About 50% of the patients were not treated for 5 years or more. The delays were greatest when symptoms began in childhood or adolescence. Even after seeing a mental health professional, most patients did not receive a diagnosis of bipolar disorder in their initial years of consultation.

CLINICAL PICTURE

The diagnostic criteria and symptom profile of pediatric bipolar depression are the same as those for adults; however, the way the symptoms are expressed varies with the developmental stage of the child (Table 4–1). For example, instead of communicating the sad feelings, children may act out and be irritable towards others, or express multiple somatic complaints, like headaches and stomachaches. Presence of specific symptoms such as psychosis, psychomotor retardation, medication-induced disinhibition/hypomania, or a family history of bipolar disorder may indicate that the depressed patient is at risk to develop bipolar disorder (Geller et al. 1994; Strober and Carlson 1982; Strober et al. 1993). Somatic complaints and thoughts of death are common. Adolescent patients may be more likely to present with rapid cycling or mixed episodes. These patients are difficult to treat and are at an increased risk for suicide (Brent

TABLE 4–1.   Clues to diagnosing bipolar illness in children

A.   **Symptoms of depression common to adults, children, and adolescents**
Depressed mood, sadness or irritable mood
Diminished interest in activities once enjoyed
Significant weight loss or weight gain
Insomnia or hypersomnia
Psychomotor agitation or retardation
Loss of energy
Feelings of worthlessness or inappropriate guilt
Difficulty focusing or concentrating
Recurrent thoughts of death or suicide

B.   **Symptoms and characteristics commonly seen in depressed children**
Somatic complaints that are vague, like headaches and stomachaches
Absences from school, school refusal, or poor academic performance
Running away or threats to run away from home
Isolating self or lack of friends
Boredom
Decreased interest in playing or interacting with friends
Substance abuse, especially alcohol or marijuana
Outbursts of shouting, complaining, unexplained irritability, or crying
Preoccupation with death or thoughts of death
Increased irritability, anger outbursts, or hostility
Reckless behavior
Relationship difficulties

C.   **Characteristics commonly suggestive of bipolar depression in children**
Family history of bipolar disorder
Early age at onset of depressive symptoms
Presence of mood congruent psychotic symptoms
Comorbid illness: conduct disorder, oppositional defiant disorder
Anhedonia
Suicidal ideations or attempts
Hospitalization, especially early age and frequency
Poorly controlled ADHD

Source.   Adapted from Benazzi 1999a, 1999b, 2003; Kuhs and Reschke 1992; Strober et al. 1993; Wozniak et al. 2001, 2002, 2004.

et al. 1988, 1993; Geller and Luby 1997). Clinically, these children are categorized as having bipolar disorder not otherwise specified (NOS) or mixed, even after a correct diagnosis of bipolar disorder.

Prepubertal Children

Depressed children are more likely to be irritable, frustrated, moody, cranky and withdrawn (Table 4–1, section B) and are less likely to report feelings of sadness or hopelessness than adolescents and adults. In most cases, the most common presentation is sadness. These children may also exhibit mixed symptoms by cycling between depression and mania/hypomania several times a day. Egeland et al. (2000) studied the prodromal symptoms most commonly reported by families on initial admission of 58 children who were later diagnosed with bipolar disorder. The most common symptoms were depressed mood (53%), increased energy (47%), decreased energy and tiredness (38%), anger outbursts (38%), and irritable mood (33%).

Luby and Mrakotsky (2003) studied the association of increased rate of switching to mania in childhood depressive disorder. These patients had an earlier age at onset of an episode of depression as well as a family history of bipolar disorder. From a pool of 174 preschoolers, ages 3.0–5.6 years, 54 of them met modified criteria for major depressive disorder. This study indicated that the group of depressed preschoolers had a greater incidence of having a family history of bipolar disorder compared with the two comparison groups. Luby and Mrakotsky also found that patients with major depressive symptoms along with a family history of bipolar disorder had a significantly higher chance of having mothers with an affective disorder. This research suggests that the studied at-risk subgroup might face both genetic and psychosocially transmitted familial risk factors. The increased restlessness and motor agitation exhibited by these children could be precursors of later mania.

Geller et al. (2001b) followed 72 children with histories of prepubertal major depression for a mean of 10 years. Thirty-five (48.6%) developed a bipolar disorder, of which 24 (33.3%) were type I. This rate of developing bipolar disorder was significantly higher than in a comparison group without childhood psychiatric illness (7.1% developed bipolar disorder in the comparison group). The difference was significant for type I, but not type II, illness. Additionally, children with prepubertal depression had a higher rate of substance abuse (30.6% vs. 10.7% in children without psychiatric illness) and suicidality (22.2% vs. 3.6%) (Geller et al. 2001b).

The difficulty in diagnosing bipolar disorder in children is exemplified in the following case:

Case 1

Samantha is a 7-year-old, white female who was admitted to the psychiatric inpatient unit for the fifth time in the last 2 years. She was admitted following explosive and destructive behavior at school and threats of suicide and self-harm—she had apparently stabbed herself with a pencil in a fit of anger. Her history indicates disinhibitive and aggressive behaviors with trials of sertaline, fluoxetine, diphenhydramine, and meth-ylphenidate. After having initially received the diagnosis of major depression, she did not respond positively to multiple psychopharma-cological trials with antidepressants. She was noted to have a good re-sponse to lithium but was noncompliant with the treatment. She has a history of being severely depressed, irritable, and has daily mood cy-cling. There is no historical evidence of mania/hypomania or any form of abuse. Her family history is positive for severe affective disorders in-cluding a diagnosis of bipolar disorder for her biological mother and grandmother.

Adolescents

The clinical presentation of adolescents is more similar to that of adults than to that of children. McGlashan (1988) and Strober et al. (1995) have reported that adolescents with bipolar disorder may have a more pro-longed early course and may be less responsive to treatment when com-pared with adults. Lewinsohn et al. (1995) reported that 61.1% of adolescents studied with bipolar disorder presented with a major or mi-nor depressive episode. Depression should be considered when a pre-viously well-functioning child performs poorly academically and in other school functions, withdraws from friends or society, or commits delinquent acts. Atypical clinical presentation is common in adoles-cents with bipolar disorder (McElroy et al. 1992). Substance abuse is commonly seen with depressive disorders in adolescents (Rao et al. 1995).

Strober et al. (1993) studied 60 hospitalized, depressed adolescents (ages 13–16 years) and found that at the 3- to 4-year follow-up, 20% of these patients had developed bipolar disorder. This was predicted by the rapid onset of depressive symptoms, psychomotor retardation, fam-ily history of bipolar disorder, medication-induced mania/hypomania, and mood-congruent psychosis. Geller et al. (1994, 2001b) also noted similar presentation in two studies.

According to Wozniak et al. (2004), children and adolescentes with bipolar depression were more likely to have comorbid psychiatric conditions, such as conduct disorder, severe oppositional and defiant disorder, agoraphobia, obsessive-compulsive disorder, and alcohol abuse, compared with children with unipolar depression. This study also found that, in adolescents, bipolar depression differed from uni-polar depression in quality and severity of symptoms, comorbid ill-ness, and family history. Depressive symptoms were severe in these children who exhibited profound anhedonia, hopelessness, and sui-cidality.

Suicide

Wozniak et al. (2004) reported a higher rate of suicidality (ideation and attempts) among adolescents with bipolar depression than among those with unipolar depression. Brent et al. (1988) found that suicide victims ($n=27$), compared with those with suicide ideation or who have made an attempt ($n=56$), were more likely to suffer from bipolar disorder with a trend toward higher comorbidity with attention-deficit/hyperactivity disorder (ADHD), a condition which is characterized by mood instability and a high degree of impulsivity.

Case 2

Ethan is a 14-year-old, white male brought to the hospital by police for assaultive behavior and suicidal ideation: he had taken a gun to school and threatened to kill himself in front of his classmates. According to his teachers, Ethan had been skipping class, getting increasingly moody, irritable, and frustrated over the past several weeks. He was noted to be extremely sensitive and to have rage episodes and crying spells without any provocation. Ethan's mother reported that he had been sleeping all the time, sometimes 12–14 hours at a stretch and his mood was always irritable and angry. He had punched several holes in the walls at home and had missed taking his medications for several days. His mother gave history of prior hospitalizations for risky and reckless behaviors (he had attempted to kill himself on several occasions). He was reported to be preoccupied with death, thoughts of suicide, and assault weapons. Ethan has a documented history of mania requiring a psychiatric hospitalization when he was 12 years old. Both Ethan and his mother admit that the depressive symptoms are severe and chronic and that they trouble Ethan more so than the manic episodes.

DIFFERENTIAL DIAGNOSIS

The overlapping symptoms of other psychiatric and medical disorders with those of pediatric bipolar depression makes it difficult to differentiate. Even when a diagnosis of bipolar disorder is made, the differentiation between the subcategories of bipolar disorder is challenging. The majority of children with this presentation are labeled as having bipolar disorder NOS or mixed state.

Attention-Deficit/Hyperactivity Disorder

The cardinal symptoms of ADHD (e.g., distractibility, impulsivity, hyperactivity, or emotional lability) are also present in bipolar disorder (Biederman et al. 1996; Carlson 1984). The differential diagnosis is difficult because these conditions frequently coexist (Kovacs and Gatsonis 1994). Geller et al. (1995), Wozniak et al. (1995), and West et al. (1995) found rates of 57%–98% of comorbid ADHD in bipolar patients. Butler et al. (1995) found a 22% rate of bipolar disorder in inpatients with ADHD.

Attention-deficit disorder (ADD) symptoms often mimic those of dysphoria/depression, especially in girls. This may create problems in making the correct diagnosis. However, ADD patients rarely complain of suicidal ideation or thoughts of death and self-harm. Furthermore, a positive family history for bipolar disorder or affective disorder in the family of those patients with ADD should raise a red flag for the treating clinician.

Schizophrenia

Some of the negative symptoms seen in schizophrenia are also seen in depression. Children with clinical presentation of bipolar disorder and psychotic mood disorders are often misdiagnosed as having schizophrenia (Ferro et al. 1994); however, their symptoms may be distinguishable by the associated mood-incongruent hallucinations and paranoia seen in patients with schizophrenia. Furthermore, patients with schizophrenia have an insidious onset and are less likely to have episodic pattern of mood changes and lack family history of bipolar disorder.

Other Conditions

In the differential diagnosis of pediatric bipolar depression, all of the following should be considered: medical illness, exposure to medications, substance abuse, and other psychiatric conditions, such as reactive attachment disorder or conduct disorder.

TREATMENT

Standardized and universally accepted treatment regimens for bipolar depression are lacking at this time. The treatment of pediatric bipolar disorder has not yet been studied sufficiently (Botteron and Geller 1995; Fetner and Geller 1992; Kafantaris 1995; Youngerman and Canino 1978). Most of the treatment options are extrapolated from adult studies or studies showing benefit for treatment of the manic phase or aggressive behavior in children.

Psychotherapy

Psychosocial interventions are critical in the management of pediatric bipolar depression, although there is no proven, superior psychotherapeutic method. Pavuluri et al. (2004b) suggested the integration of cognitive-behavioral therapy and interpersonal therapy to help patients and families deal with their negative cognitions. A manual-driven, adjunctive, multiple-family, group treatment for adolescents (ages 8–12 years) with bipolar depression was attempted by Fristad et al. (2002). The results and impact of this treatment on the adolescents are still pending. Although lacking in documented scientific merit as a proven treatment for bipolar disorder, cognitive-behavioral therapy has shown promise—especially for adolescents with bipolar depression (see Chapter 10, "Psychological Interventions in Bipolar Depression").

Pharmacotherapy

There is a paucity of studies involving children with diagnoses of bipolar disorders. As of now no standardized, scientific research data exist for the treatment of pediatric bipolar depression. Several agents have been clinically tried with limited success in controlling this complex illness. There is a great need for clinical trials examining the safety and efficacy of psychotropic medications in the treatment of bipolar depression in children.

Lithium

The U.S. Food and Drug Administration has approved lithium for treatment of bipolar disorder in individuals age 12 years or older; adult studies indicate significant effect size for lithium (Schou 1968; Strober et al. 1990). Only a few studies have examined the efficacy of lithium in children from both the prepubertal and adolescent population. Available data indicate lithium is both safe and effective in youths and can be prescribed in a manner similar to that for the adult population (Strober et al. 1995; Weller et al. 1986). El-Mallakh et al. (1993) suggested that very young children would require higher serum lithium levels to get adequate response. The benefit of lithium in depressed children at risk for bipolar disorder was observed in a double-blind, placebo-controlled study by Geller et al. (Fetner and Geller 1992; Geller et al. 1994). Similarly, DeLong and Aldershof (1987) described significant improvement with lithium in children with severe depression who exhibit neurovegetative symptoms.

Anti-Epileptic Agents

Several studies in adults and adolescents have shown the significant benefit of anti-epileptic agents, like carbamazepine and valproate (Hsu 1986; Kowatch et al. 2000; Woolston 1999). However, these studies were primarily for patients with classic manic episodes or mixed episodes—no significant benefit was noted in regards to pediatric bipolar depression. Adult studies have indicated a potential benefit in bipolar depression from lamotrigine (Calabrese et al. 1999; Fatemi et al. 1997); however, children below the age of 16 years may be particularly vulnerable to development of worrisome rash or Stevens-Johnson syndrome with this agent—this has limited the examination of lamotrigine in children.

Selective Serotonin Reuptake Inhibitors

Antidepressant medications are widely prescribed in children and adolescents. Prior to the diagnosis of bipolar disorder, most of these patients have been misdiagnosed as having major depression. They have been treated with antidepressants, with subsequent disinhibitive behavior outbursts and manic/hypomanic inductions. A naturalistic chart review of 59 youths (ages 10.8±3.7 years, range 3.5–17; 83% were boys) from an outpatient psychopharmacology clinic with DSM-III-R diagnosis of bipolar disorder was reported by Biederman et al. (2000). These children were followed for up to 4 years. The researchers applied multivariate statistics to model the probability of relapse or improvement at each clinical visit. This analysis showed that the serotonin-specific antidepressants were associated with an increased rate of improvement of bipolar depression (relative risk 6.7 [1.9–23.6], $P=0.003$), but a significantly greater probability of relapse of mania (relative risk 3.0 [1.2–7.8], $P=0.02$). The study also indicated that the antidepressant-associated manic induction documented in adults may also occur in children.

Cicero et al. (2003) reported that children treated with antidepressants received the diagnosis for bipolar disorder earlier (ages 10.7 ±3.05 years) than children never exposed to these medications (ages 12.7±4.3 years; one-tailed $t=-1.33$, $df=22$, $P=0.099$, power=0.93). DelBello et al. (2001) found that children receiving stimulant medication had an earlier age at onset of bipolar disorder (ages 10.7±3.9 years, $n=21$) than children who did not receive stimulants (ages 13.9±3.7 years, $n=13$, $P=0.03$). This difference was not explained by concomitant ADHD, because the age at onset of bipolar illness in children with or without ADHD was not different (ages 12.0±4.2 vs. 11.7±4.0 years, respectively, $P=0.6$). However, Cicero et al. (2003) reported a relatively greater safety with stimulants compared with antidepressants.

Clinical experience indicates that a child with bipolar disorder will commonly present to the medical professional with depressive symptoms. The U.S. Food and Drug Administration has recently implemented a "black box warning" about the risk of suicidality with antidepressant use in adolescents and children. Some experts have opined that the increase in suicidal ideation with antidepressants may be due to destabilization of unrecognized bipolar disorder in children. Antidepressants are effective (El-Mallakh and Karippot 2002) but should be used with caution in patients presenting with symptoms of severe depression. A longitudinal symptom history and a thorough family history for the evidence of bipolar disorder will help with decision making and better management of this complex illness.

SUMMARY

Pediatric bipolar depression is increasingly recognized in the scientific literature. A great deal of debate exists about the clinical presentation, core symptoms, and treatment options. There is a monumental need for research of bipolar depression in children and adolescents. Randomized clinical trials and standardized treatment algorithm studies will provide more effective treatment recommendations in the future.

REFERENCES

Angold A: Childhood and adolescent depression. I. Epidemiological and aetiological aspects. Br J Psychiatry 152:601–611, 1988a

Angold A: Childhood and adolescent depression. II: Research in clinical populations. Br J Psychiatry 153:476–492, 1988b

Benazzi F: Bipolar II versus unipolar chronic depression: a 312-case study. Compr Psychiatry 40:418–421, 1999a

Benazzi F: Chronic atypical major depressive episode in private practice: unipolar and bipolar II. Acta Psychiatr Scand 100:418–423, 1999b

Biederman J, Faraone SV, Milberger S, et al: Predictors of persistence and remission of ADHD: results from a four-year prospective follow-up study of ADHD children. J Am Acad Child Adolesc Psychiatry 35:343–351, 1996

Biederman J, Mick E, Spencer TJ, et al: Therapeutic dilemmas in the pharmacotherapy of bipolar depression in the young. J Child Adolesc Psychiatry 10:185–192, 2000

Botteron KN, Geller B: Pharmacologic treatment of childhood and adolescent mania. Child Adolesc Psychiatr Clin N Am 4:283–304, 1995

Brent DA, Perper JA, Goldstein CE, et al: Risk factors for adolescent suicide. A comparison of adolescent suicide victims with suicidal inpatients. Arch Gen Psychiatry 45:581–588, 1988

Brent DA, Perper JA, Moritz G, et al: Psychiatric risk factors for adolescent suicide: a case-control study. J Am Acad Child Adolesc Psychiatry 32:521–529, 1993

Butler SF, Arredondo DE, McCloskey V: Affective comorbidity in children and adolescents with attention deficit hyperactivity disorder. Ann Clin Psychiatry 7:51–55, 1995

Calabrese JR, Rapport DJ, Kimmel SE, et al: Controlled trials in bipolar I depression: focus on switch rates and efficacy. Eur Neuropsychopharmacol 9 (suppl 4):S109–S112, 1999

Carlson GA: Classification issues of bipolar disorders in childhood. Psychiatr Rev 2:273–285, 1984

Cicero D, El-Mallakh RS, Holman J, et al: Antidepressant exposure in children diagnosed with bipolar disorder. Psychiatry 66:317–322, 2003

DelBello MP, Soutullo CA, Hendricks W, et al: Prior stimulant treatment in adolescents with bipolar disorder: association with age at onset. Bipolar Disord 3:53–57, 2001

DeLong GR, Aldershof AL: Long-term experience with lithium treatment in childhood: correlation with clinical diagnosis. J Am Acad Child Adolesc Psychiatry 26:389–394, 1987

Egeland JA, Hostetter AM, Pauls DL, et al: Prodromal symptoms before onset of manic-depressive disorder suggested by first hospital admission histories. J Am Acad Child Adolesc Psychiatry 39:1245–1252, 2000

El-Mallakh RS, Karippot A: Use of antidepressants to treat depression in bipolar disorder. Psychiatric Serv 53:580–584, 2002

El-Mallakh RS, Barrett JL, Wyatt RJ: The Na,K-ATPase hypothesis for bipolar disorder: implications of normal development. J Child Adolesc Psychopharmacol 3:37–52, 1993

Fatemi SH, Rapport DJ, Calabrese JR, et al: Lamotrigine in rapid-cycling bipolar disorder. J Clin Psychiatry 58:522–527, 1997

Ferro T, Carlson GA, Grayson P, et al: Depressive disorders: distinctions in Children. J Am Acad Child Adolesc Psychiatry 33:664–670, 1994

Fetner HH, Geller B: Lithium and tricyclic antidepressants. Psychiatr Clin North Am 15:223–224, 1992

Fleming JE, Offord DR: Epidemiology of childhood depressive disorders: a critical review. J Am Acad Child Adolesc Psychiatry 29:571–580, 1990

Fristad MA, Goldberg-Arnold JS, Gavazzi SM: Multifamily psychoeducation groups (MFPG) for families of children with bipolar disorder. Bipolar Disord 4:254–262, 2002

Geller B, Luby J: Child and adolescent bipolar disorder: a review of the past 10 years. J Am Acad Child Adolesc Psychiatry 36:1168–1176, 1997

Geller B, Fox LW, Clark KA: Rate and predictors of prepubertal bipolarity during follow-up of 6- to 12-year-old depressed children. J Am Acad Child Adolesc Psychiatry 33:461–468, 1994

Geller B, Sun K, Zimerman B, et al: Complex and rapid cycling in bipolar children and adolescents: a preliminary study. J Affect Disord 34:259–268, 1995

Geller B, Craney JL, Bolhofner K, et al: One-year recovery and relapse rates of children with a prepubertal and early adolescent bipolar disorder phenotype. Am J Psychiatry 158:303–305, 2001a

Geller B, Zimerman B, Williams M, et al: Bipolar disorder at prospective follow-up of adults who had prepubertal major depressive disorder. Am J Psychiatry 158:125–127, 2001b

Hirschfeld RM, Calabrese JR, Weissman MM, et al: Screening for bipolar disorder in the community. J Clin Psychiatry 64:53–59, 2003

Hsu LK: Lithium-resistant adolescent mania. J Am Acad Child Adolesc Psychiatry 25:280–283, 1986

Kafantaris V: Treatment of bipolar disorder in children and adolescents. J Am Acad Child Adolesc Psychiatry 34:732–741, 1995

Kowatch RA, Suppes T, Carmody TJ, et al: Effect size of lithium, divalproex sodium, and carbamazepine in children and adolescents with bipolar disorder. J Am Acad Child Adolesc Psychiatry 39:713–720, 2000

Kovacs M: Presentation and course of major depressive disorder during childhood and later years of the life span. J Am Acad Child Adolesc Psychiatry 35:705–715, 1996

Kovacs M, Gatsonis C: Secular trends in age at onset of major depressive disorder in a clinical sample of children. J Psychiatr Res 28:319–329, 1994

Kuhs H, Reschke D: Psychomotor activity in unipolar and bipolar depressive patients. Psychopathology 25:109–116, 1992

Lewinsohn PM, Hops H, Roberts RE, et al: Adolescent psychopathology: I. prevalence and incidence of depression and other DSM-III-R disorders in high school students. J Abnorm Psychol 102:133–144, 1993; erratum 102:517, 1993

Lewinsohn PM, Klein DN, Seeley JR: Bipolar disorders in a community sample of older adolescents: prevalence, phenomenology, comorbidity, and course. J Am Acad Child Adolesc Psychiatry 34:454–463, 1995

Lish JD, Dime-Meenan S, Whybrow PC, et al: The national depressive and manic-depressive association (DMDA) survey of bipolar members. J Affect Disord 31:281–294, 1994

Luby JL, Mrakotsky C: Depressed preschoolers with bipolar family history: a group at high risk for later switching to mania? J Child Adolesc Psychiatry 13:187–197, 2003

McElroy SL, Keck PE Jr, Pope HG Jr, et al: Clinical and research implications of the diagnosis of dysphoric or mixed mania or hypomania. Am J Psychiatry 149:1633–1644, 1992

McGlashan TH: Adolescent versus adult onset of mania. Am J Psychiatry 145:221–223, 1988

Pavuluri MN, Henry DB, Devineni B, et al : Child Mania Rating Scale (CMRS): development, reliability and validity. Biol Psychiatry 55:S84, 2004a

Pavuluri MN, Henry DB, Devineni B, et al : A pharmacotherapy algorithm for stabilization and maintenance of pediatric bipolar disorder. J Am Acad Child Adolesc Psychiatry 43:859–867, 2004b

Rao U, Ryan ND, Birmaher B, et al: Unipolar depression in adolescents: clinical outcome in adulthood. J Am Acad Child Adolesc Psychiatry 34:566–578, 1995

Raskin A, Boothe H, Reatig N, et al: Initial response to drugs in depressive illness and psychiatric and community adjustment a year later. Psychol Med 8:71–79, 1978

Sanchez L, Hagino O, Weller E, et al: Bipolarity in children. Psychiatr Clin North Am 22:629–648, 1999

Schou M: Lithium in psychiatric therapy and prophylaxis. J Psychiatr Res 6:67–95, 1968

Strober M, Carlson G: Predictors of bipolar illness in adolescents with major depression: a follow-up investigation. Adolesc Psychiatry 10:299–319, 1982

Strober M, Morrell W, Lampert C, et al: Relapse following discontinuation of lithium maintenance therapy in adolescents with bipolar I illness: a naturalistic study. Am J Psychiatry 147:457–461, 1990

Strober M, Lampert C, Schmidt S, et al: The course of major depressive disorder in adolescents: I. Recovery and risk of manic switching in a follow-up of psychotic and non-psychotic subtypes. J Am Acad Child Adolesc Psychiatry 32:34–42, 1993

Strober M, Schmidt-Lackner S, Freeman R, et al: Recovery and relapse in adolescents with bipolar affective illness: a five-year naturalistic, prospective follow-up. J Am Acad Child Adolesc Psychiatry 34:724–731, 1995

Weissman MM, Warner V, John K, et al: Delusional depression and bipolar spectrum: evidence for a possible association from a family study of children. Neuropsychopharmacology 1:257–264, 1988

Weller EB, Weller RA: Assessing depression in prepubertal children. Hillside J Clin Psychiatry 8:193–201, 1986a

Weller EB, Weller RA: Clinical aspects of childhood depression. Pediatr Ann 15:843–847, 1986b

Weller EB, Weller RA, Fristad MA: Lithium dosage guide for prepubertal children: a preliminary report. J Am Acad Child Psychiatry 25:92–95, 1986

West SA, Strakowski SM, Sax KW, et al: The comorbidity of attention-deficit hyperactivity disorder in adolescent mania: potential diagnostic and treatment implications. Psychopharmacol Bull 31:347–351, 1995

Woolston JL: Case study: carbamazepine treatment of juvenile-onset bipolar disorder. J Am Acad Child Adolesc Psychiatry 38:335–338, 1999

Wozniak J, Biederman J, Kiely K, et al: Mania-like symptoms suggestive of childhood-onset bipolar disorder in clinically referred children. J Am Acad Child Adolesc Psychiatry 34:867–976, 1995

Wozniak J, Biederman J, Faraone SV, et al: Heterogeneity of childhood conduct disorder: further evidence of a subtype of conduct disorder linked to bipolar disorder. J Affect Disord 64:121–131, 2001

Wozniak J, Biederman J, Monuteaux MC, et al: Parsing the comorbidity between bipolar disorder and anxiety disorders: a familial risk analysis. J Child Adolesc Psychopharmacol 12:101–111, 2002

Wozniak J, Spencer T, Biederman J, et al: The clinical characteristics of unipolar vs. bipolar major depression in ADHD youth. J Affect Disord 82 (suppl 1):S59–S69, 2004

Youngerman J, Canino IA: Lithium carbonate use in children and adolescents: a survey of the literature. Arch Gen Psychiatry 35:216–224, 1978

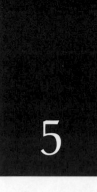

5

SUICIDE IN
BIPOLAR DEPRESSION

Michael J. Ostacher, M.D., M.P.H.
Polina Eidelman, B.A.

> Dearest, I feel certain I am going mad again. I feel
> we can't go through another of those terrible
> times. And I shan't recover this time. I begin to
> hear voices, and I can't concentrate. So I am do-
> ing what seems the best thing to do.
>
> —*Virginia Woolf, suicide note*

PERHAPS THE MOST LETHAL mental illness, with a suicide rate for untreated cases 30 times that found in the general population, bipolar disorder presents an enormous challenge to patients, families, and treaters.
The lifetime rate of suicide in bipolar disorder has been estimated to be
as high as 19%, equaling (and perhaps surpassing) that of major depressive disorder. While the majority of suicides, like that of Virginia Woolf,
occur during the depressed phase of the illness, many occur during periods of mixed or even manic symptoms. There are many risk factors for
suicide in this illness, the most prominent being early onset of mood
symptoms, recent diagnosis and young age, family history of suicide,
comorbidity of anxiety disorders and substance use disorders (includ-

117

ing nicotine), the presence of physical and sexual abuse in childhood and adulthood, and a history of prior suicide attempts. Engagement in treatment and adherence to pharmacological treatment (especially lithium) may reduce suicide risk. Coordinated treatment planning with the patient, the patient's family, and persons with whom the patient has significant relationships may provide a means for identifying risk and avoiding suicidal behavior.

EPIDEMIOLOGY

The lifetime prevalence of all bipolar disorders (bipolar I and II combined) is approximately 2.1%, and for bipolar I disorder alone it is 0.8%. Typically, bipolar disorder is imagined primarily as a disorder characterized by mood elevation, yet long-term studies of clinical cohorts suggest that the disorder is primarily characterized by depression. Both bipolar I and II patients spend half of their lives ill, with most of those days spent depressed (Judd et al. 2002, 2003). In the context of illnesses with vast periods of depression, it is easily understood that the risk for suicide attempts and completed suicides would be inordinately high.

Although it is unclear whether the rate of suicide in bipolar disorder is higher than that for unipolar depression, several studies suggest that it is. For example, data from the Epidemiologic Catchment Area (ECA) Study reported by Chen and Dilsaver (1996) show lifetime rates of suicide attempts of 29.2% in bipolar disorder, 15.9% in unipolar major depression, and 4.2% in all other DSM-III Axis I disorders combined. They found an odds ratio of suicides in bipolar compared with unipolar of 2.0 ($P<0.0001$).

While there is consensus that the rate of suicide in bipolar disorder is disproportionately high, it has been difficult to ascertain it with precision. Suicide rates in psychiatric disorders are frequently estimated using studies of clinical populations; this will generally lead to overestimations of rates of completed suicides for the illness as a whole, as patients who are more ill are more likely to make suicide attempts. Goodwin and Jamison (1990), for instance, estimated the lifetime risk of mortality from suicide for bipolar patients to be 18.9% by examining all causes of death from subjects with manic-depressive illness in 30 studies published between 1936 and 1988. As this represents a severely ill group with bipolar disorder, it likely overestimates the risk of suicide from bipolar disorder as a whole. One of the most cited papers on suicide in affective disorders is that of Guze and Robins in 1970, where the lifetime risk of death by suicide due to depressive disorders was estimated to be 15%.

The Guze and Robins finding has been criticized as not being generalizable to the general population on several grounds, most commonly because subjects were not actually followed over their entire lifespan, and since suicide accounts for a larger percentage of overall mortality in younger populations, the prevalence of suicide was markedly overestimated. Blair-West et al. (1997) accounted for this in major depression by adding the lifetime risk for suicide in each age group, and concluded that the rate is 2.5%. After adjustment for an estimated rate of 40% for underreporting of suicide, the lifetime risk climbs to 3.5%. Similarly, Inskip et al. (1998) recalculated the lifetime risk of death from affective disorders using computer modeling techniques to take into account the fact that subjects are not followed until the entire cohort has died and that suicide is a disproportionately high cause of death in younger patients. They thereby estimated that the lifetime risk of death from affective disorders was approximately 6%, compared with 4% for schizophrenia and 7% for alcohol dependence

Sampling bias may also overestimate the suicide rate. Bostwick and Pankrantz (2000) contend that the use of proportionate mortality prevalence (i.e., the percentage of all deaths attributable to suicide) overestimates the lifetime prevalence of suicide. Instead, they propose that case fatality prevalence (i.e., the percentage of cases of depression who die by suicide) is a more accurate measure of the actual rate. Rather than the 15% risk claimed by Guze and Robins, their analysis found that the risk of suicide for all patients with affective disorders—both inpatients and outpatients—was 2.2%. This was four times the rate in the non–affectively ill population (0.5%): higher in patients who had been hospitalized for severe depression, but considerably lower than previous estimates.

Markedly elevated rates of suicide have been found in clinical cohorts followed longitudinally. In a remarkable study of 406 patients followed from 1959 to 1995, Angst and Preisig (1995) found that 11% of the sample had committed suicide. Diagnostic subtype did not differentiate suicide rates. It is not answered whether this sample was biased by severity of illness, whether the study compared all patients affected with these disorders, or whether advances in the treatment of depression or bipolar disorder would have prevented any suicides.

In a naturalistic study of 2,395 hospital admissions for unipolar or bipolar disorder, the lethality of suicide attempts was higher in patients with bipolar disorder, and this may partly explain the increased rates of completed suicide compared with other disorders (Raja and Azzoni 2004). Whether for all Axis I disorders suicide is greatest in bipolar disorder may be unclear; it is nonetheless the case that the mortality rate in bipolar disorder is strikingly high, compared with the general population.

RISK FACTORS FOR SUICIDE

Phase of Illness

The frequency and duration of depressive symptoms and episodes is one factor in the high incidence of suicide and suicide attempts in bipolar disorder. In a study of 31 suicides of people with bipolar disorder, nearly 80% occurred during an episode of depression, 11% while in a mixed state, and 9% while the person was recovering from a episode of psychotic mania (Isometsa et al. 1994). We can therefore conclude that depression, whether during a major depressive or mixed episode, is associated with suicide. Dilsaver et al. (1994) reported that whereas suicidal ideation was rare in pure mania (occurring in 1 of 49 subjects studied), 55% of the patients with mixed mania had suicidal ideation, and that this difference was significant ($P=0.0001$).

Additional observations support the notion that it is depression that puts patients with bipolar disorder at risk of suicide. Those with a course of illness characterized predominantly by mania or mania with mild depression were found by Angst et al. (2004) to have a lower suicidality rate and chronicity compared with those whose course was one of more severe depression.

It does appear that manic states may put specific people at risk for suicide, in large part because of the concurrent presence of depressive symptoms. Simpson and Jamison (1999) suggested that euphoric mania may be "more of a research concept that a clinical reality" (p. 53) in that severe mania rarely is without depressive or dysphoric symptoms. Cassidy and Carroll (2001), for instance, found that while dysphoric mood, anxiety, lability, guilt, and suicidality were more common in mixed episodes, these symptoms were also present to a significant degree in "pure" manic states. In a study of 91 inpatients with mixed and manic states, Strakowski et al. (1996) found that while suicidal ideation was more likely to be present in mixed versus manic patients, the severity of depression was a more powerful predictor of suicidal ideation. In a logistical regression model, depressive symptoms predicted suicidality whether or not the patient met criteria for a depressive (and therefore, mixed) episode.

Clinical Course

Severity of illness appears to be associated with suicide. First episodes requiring hospitalization may be particularly high risk. The time immediately after hospital admission and immediately after discharge appears to be a particularly vulnerable period for suicide. Hoyer et al. (2004) examined the characteristics of all first hospitalizations for affective disorder in Denmark between 1973 and 1993, finding that 3,141 of 53,466 patients committed suicide (6%), and that the suicide risk was highest on the day following discharge and the day following admission. The risk declined over time, remaining high for 6 months following discharge. Interestingly, the risk associated with time after discharge declined with increasing duration of illness, supporting the notion that suicide risk is highest early in the course of affective illnesses, including in bipolar disorder.

Individuals appear to be most at risk for suicidality following their index affective episode, regardless of episode polarity (Fagiolini et al. 2004; Roy-Byrne et al. 1988). Baldessarini et al. (1999), in an analysis of 104 suicide attempts considered over a period of 40 years, demonstrated that over 50% occurred within 7.5 years of the initial affective episode. It is also important to note that, within this same sample, the time to suicide attempt was well before the time to lithium maintenance treatment. It follows that younger patients and those with an earlier age at onset may also find themselves at greater risk for suicidality as a result of the lag in time between illness onset and appropriate treatment. This also demonstrates the inherent dangers involved in misdiagnosing unipolar depression for bipolar individuals following an index depressive episode. These individuals may not be represented in current research as a result and may instead be victims of misdiagnosis and inappropriate clinical care.

Fagiolini et al. (2004) reported that in a cohort of 175 patients with bipolar disorder, suicide attempts tended to occur at a relatively young age and in the early part of the patients' illnesses. A history of suicide was also associated with a greater number of prior episodes, higher depression scores at entry, and higher body mass index (BMI) (Fagiolini et al. 2004). Tsai et al. (2002) found that in Chinese patients with bipolar disorder, suicide tended to occur in the first 7 to 12 years of illness, and the risk was greatest prior to age 35.

In addition to young age being a factor in suicide attempts, the age at onset of bipolar disorder is also associated with later suicide and is commonly seen as one measure of illness severity. Early-onset and very early-onset bipolar disorder predisposes patients to a more chronic and severe course of illness and predicts a greater likelihood of making a suicide attempt. This assumption is echoed in suicide research, in which an earlier age at bipolar onset tends to be associated with a greater risk of suicidality in bipolar patients (Coryell et al. 2003; Fagiolini et al. 2004; Goodwin and Jamison 1990; Guze and Robins 1970; Levine et al. 2001).

Therefore, it is likely that younger bipolar patients may be a high-risk group for suicide attempts and completion.

Early Illness Onset

In a study of 1,000 bipolar subjects, Perlis et al. (2004) reported that 55.3% of subjects had onset of illness prior to age 19, and that these patients were more likely to have comorbid anxiety and substance use disorders, less euthymic time, more episodes of illness, and were more likely to have made a suicide attempt.

In a sample of 320 bipolar I and bipolar II patients, Carter et al. (2003) found that subjects with an early age at onset (defined as earlier than age 18 years) had a more complex illness course and presented a number of additional conditions we perceive as risk factors for suicide. Specifically, the early-age-at-onset group had more frequent suicidal ideation, more frequent suicide attempts, a greater number of Axis I comorbidities, more frequent comorbid substance use disorders, and were more likely to be rapid cycling. These factors may create independent, additional burdens on the patient, may be indications of a more complex and treatment-resistant illness manifestation, or may be a consequence of early misdiagnosis and consequent, suboptimal treatment. In any case, earlier bipolar onset appears to compound suicide risk, and greater clinical vigilance with younger bipolar patients seems warranted.

Rapid Cycling

The DSM-IV-TR defines rapid cycling as four discrete episodes of mania or depression occurring within 1 year. However, the actual appearance of rapid cycling in bipolar disorder can be quite varied, and research surrounding rapid cycling (including research focusing on suicidality) remains inconsistent. While the prevalence of rapid cycling in bipolar disorder is unclear and may be difficult to diagnose, it appears that its identification is necessary for effective suicide prevention.

In a sample of 603 bipolar individuals, MacKinnon et al. (2003) found patients with rapid cycling to be significantly more likely than non–rapid cyclers to have attempted suicide (42% vs. 27% respectively). Coryell et al. (2003) also found rapid-cycling bipolar disorder to be associated with more serious suicide attempts, although it was not associated with a greater number of completed suicides. Thus, there appears to be a significant additional burden on the patient as a result of the rapid cycling that increases vulnerability to suicidality. This potential susceptibility may rest in an underlying aspect of rapid-cycling bipolar disorder that leads to a generally more complicated illness course. As an example, we may consider MacKinnon et al.'s (2003) case-controlled examination, which found rapid cycling to be associated with an earlier age at onset, higher psychiatric comorbidity, more substance and alcohol abuse, and suicidality.

Whereas the previously mentioned studies demonstrate an added risk, others, such as that of Wu and Dunner (1993), did not find a higher rate of suicide in rapid cyclers when compared to non–rapid cyclers. Slama et al. (2004) also failed to find an association between rapid cycling and suicide attempts in a French sample. However, inconsistency in suicide research is likely to be a result of the difficulties of defining and identifying rapid cycling in both research and clinical practice: because of the variety of measures and primary hypotheses of the previously mentioned studies, operational definitions and measurements of rapid cycling may vary. One result of this may be the misinterpretation of a distinct mixed episode as a presentation of rapid cycling. Consequently, as with almost all factors researched with respect to rapid cycling, the impact of rapid cycling on suicidality is not eminently clear. Nevertheless, it appears that whether or not it has a direct impact on suicidality, rapid cycling is a more complicated manifestation of bipolar disorder and requires formidable clinical management for the prophylaxis of suicidality.

Psychosis

It does not appear that psychosis raises the risk of suicide in bipolar illness. Angst and Preisig (1995) found in their Zurich cohort that the presence of schizophrenic symptoms did not have a differential impact on suicide rates. Grunebaum et al. (2001) reported that the presence of delusions in 429 subjects with schizophrenia, unipolar depression, and bipolar disorder did not correlate with whether they had suicidal ideation or had made a suicide attempt. Tsai et al. (2002) reported that in a cohort of Chinese patients, mood-congruent psychotic symptoms at the onset of illness were in fact associated with reduced risk of having made a suicide attempt.

COMORBIDITY AND SUICIDE

Comorbid psychiatric and substance use disorders are overrepresented in bipolar disorder (Brieger et al. 2003; Kessler et al. 1994, 2005; Regier et al. 1990; Simon et al. 2004; Strakowski et al. 1992). Many of these comorbidities are associated with a more difficult course of illness and with increased suicidality (Feinman and Dunner 1996; McElroy et al. 2001). In a clinical cohort of bipolar II patients in Spain, those with any comorbid condition fared far worse than those without: patients with comorbid conditions, primarily personality disorders and substance use disorders, were more likely to experience suicidal ideation (74% vs. 24%) and attempt suicide (45% vs. 5%) (Vieta et al. 2000). Although this sample is likely not representative of the illness as a whole, it does underscore the importance of evaluating comorbid conditions in bipolar disorder. We will examine the impact of several comorbid conditions on suicidality.

Anxiety Disorders

Comorbid anxiety and anxiety disorders appear to be associated with increased suicidal behavior in bipolar disorder. Simon et al. (2004) found that a history of an anxiety disorder was an independent risk factor for a more severe and debilitative course of bipolar illness, and brought on higher risk of attempting suicide (odds ratio=2.45, 95% CI=1.4–4.2). Anxiety disorders were highly prevalent in this study, with a lifetime history of an anxiety disorder in 51.2% of the sample. A current anxiety disorder was present in 30.5% of subjects.

Henry et al. (2003) did not find such an association in a smaller sample of 318 subjects with bipolar disorder. Only 24% of this sample had a lifetime anxiety disorder, and there was no increase in suicide attempts in the subjects with a history of an anxiety disorder. This sample may not have had enough statistical power to find such a difference, and their negative finding may represent a type II error (i.e., failing to find a difference when one actually exists).

A high level of lifetime panic symptoms appears to be associated with both suicidal ideation, increased depression, and a much delayed time to recover from an index mood episode in subjects with bipolar I disorder (Frank et al. 2002). They postulate that panic spectrum symptoms in patients with bipolar disorder represent a high-risk group, even if they do not meet DSM-IV-TR syndromal criteria for panic disorder. The delay to recovery is striking, with the high-panic group taking 44 weeks to recover from an acute mood episode compared with 17 weeks in the low-panic group.

Alcohol and Substance Use Disorders

Substance and alcohol abuse present a clinical challenge in the treatment of any psychiatric illness. For bipolar patients, a comorbid alcohol use disorder (AUD) or substance use disorder (SUD) not only may complicate treatment and illness course (Feinman and Dunner 1996) but also may place the patient at greater risk for suicidality. Suicide risk in alcohol or substance abusing bipolar patients has been found to be up to twice that of bipolar patients without an AUD (Morrison 1974; Tondo et al. 1999).

More recent studies of comorbid SUDs or AUDs in bipolar patients have also demonstrated an increase in suicide risk associated with substance and alcohol abuse (Dalton et al. 2003; Hoyer et al. 2004). SUD and AUD comorbidity may be particularly damaging in bipolar disorder and may reveal a unique factor of the disorder. The added suicide risk observed in bipolar patients with comorbid SUDs or AUDs may not be present in unipolar patients (Hoyer et al. 2004). Comparisons of suicide risk associated with comorbid AUDs versus that associated with comorbid SUDs have not yielded a clear difference. Dalton et al. (2003) demonstrated that drug use may present greater risk than alcohol use, with a twofold increase in suicide risk for bipolar patients with comorbid substance abuse. However, Tondo et al. (1999) did not find a similar difference. Additionally, they suggested that not all substances are associated with greater suicidality; they specify polysubstance abuse, heroin, cocaine, and tobacco abuse as additional risk factors, but note that marijuana and hallucinogens may not be as dangerous.

Because early age at illness onset has also been identified as a risk factor for suicidality in bipolar disorder, young bipolar patients with comorbid alcohol or substance use disorders may form a group that is in particular need of vigilant observation and aggressive clinical intervention. In a longitudinal, case-controlled study of 96 bipolar adolescents, Kelly, Cornelius, and Lynch (2002) demonstrate that those with comorbid SUDs are at greater risk for suicidality. A comorbid diagnosis of conduct disorder (which diagnostically shares several characteristics with both a SUD and a bipolar diagnosis) is an additional predictor.

Nicotine use and dependence is increasingly recognized as being associated with suicide in bipolar disorder. In a cohort of subjects with unipolar and bipolar disorders followed prospectively after an episode of major depression, smoking was amongst the three most powerful predictors of a future suicide attempt, and was additive with the other two: a history of a suicide attempt and severity of depressive symptoms (Oquendo et al. 2004). This association between nicotine use and suicide is present across several major mental illnesses, and may be related to lower brain serotonin function (Malone et al. 2003). The direction of the relationship between smoking and suicide and whether it is causal is unknown. It would be important to understand whether nicotine use predisposes patients to more dire outcomes, because early intervention to targeted at-risk youth may improve the course of mood disorders.

It is clear that AUDs and SUDs complicate treatment; however, they may also be an indication of a more complex illness course, illness severity, and underlying risk factors for suicidality. Potentially, these underlying difficulties may lead the patient to abuse alcohol or substances and to contemplate suicide. In this manner, comorbid SUDs and AUDs may be perceived as markers of severity in the same vein as age at onset. Although the direction of causality cannot possibly be demonstrated, SUDs and AUDs are clearly associated with increased suicide risk and require added vigilance in clinical care.

Eating Disorders

Eating disorders, while not as common of a comorbidity in bipolar disorder as substance use or anxiety disorders, is overrepresented in bipolar disorder (Krishnan 2005). In an inpatient sample there was an association between bipolar illness and eating disorders and 32% of the patients had a history of suicide attempts and self-injurious behavior (Stein et al. 2004). While rates of suicides and suicide attempts is high in patients with eating disorders, there is not enough data currently available to know whether the presence of an eating disorder in patients with bipolar disorder increases the suicide risk compared with patients without eating disorders (Corcos et al. 2002).

Personality Disorders

In the Stanley Foundation Bipolar Network study of bipolar disorder, Leverich et al. (2003) reported that cluster B personality disorders were associated with a history of suicide attempts in 648 outpatients with bipolar disorder. Prior suicide, in a hierarchical logistic regression, was associated with sexual abuse history, isolation, hospitalizations for depression, and suicidal ideation while depressed, in addition to personality disorders. The strong association that they found with sexual abuse is striking, indicating that it may be that these patients are much more at risk of personality disorders and a more chronic bipolar course (Brodsky et al. 1997).

Medical Comorbidity

Although there is a paucity of research assessing suicide risk in bipolar patients with comorbid physical illnesses, several epidemiological and treatment studies show comorbid medical illnesses to be associated with more complex bipolar course (Berglund and Nilsson 1987; Fagiolini et al. 2004; Vieta et al. 1992). Berglund and Nilsson (1987) also found a higher mortality rate in bipolar patients with a concomitant physical illness; the same increase in mortality was not present in unipolar participants.

Fagiolini et al. (2004) found obesity (as measured by BMI) to be associated with a more severe and complex illness course and an increased suicide risk in bipolar I patients. Obese, bipolar I patients had a greater number of past depressive and manic episodes, "presented a more severe index episode," and were more likely to relapse after the index episode was treated. Although additional research for suicide risk associated with specific comorbid physical illnesses is needed, a general proclivity to medical comorbidities appears to indicate greater suicide risk and a need to address both the psychiatric and the physical conditions.

Low cholesterol levels may be linked to suicide and aggression, but there is conflicting data in the literature on bipolar disorder regarding the cholesterol level of suicide attempters (Zureik et al. 1996). Bocchetta et al. (2001) observed that men with affective disorder treated with lithium and with fasting cholesterol in the lowest quartile were more likely to have a history of suicide attempts or a first-degree relative who had committed suicide than subjects whose cholesterol was in the highest quartile. Tsai et al. (2002), however, reported no association between fasting cholesterol and completed suicides in a Chinese cohort compared with living controls.

GENETIC VULNERABILITY

While bipolar disorder and suicidality appear to be heritable, it is unclear whether the vulnerability to suicide is inherited through bipolar disorder or instead through a shared genetic predisposition that is independent of bipolar disorder (or any other shared psychiatric illness, such as unipolar depression or anxiety disorders). The serotonin (5-HT$_{2A}$) receptor is of particular interest because of the association between serotonin and suicide, but research is sparse and conflicting (likely because of the small sample sizes in recent genetic studies and because suicide is a rare event) (Moffitt et al. 1998; Oquendo et al. 2003). Polymorphisms in the 5-HT$_{2A}$ receptor gene may play a role in the genetic susceptibility to bipolar disorder: Bonnier et al. (2002) found a higher-than-expected proportion of bipolar subjects with the A allele for the 5-HT$_{2A}$ receptor gene who had not made a suicide attempt, but others have found no association (Massat et al. 2000; Ni et al. 2002; Tut et al. 2000). Nonetheless, endophenotypes—allelic variations associated with a clinical phenotype—may be found in which the risk for suicide may be elevated in bipolar disorder.

TREATMENT INTERVENTIONS

Psychopharmacologic Interventions: Potential Prophylactic Effects

Appropriate maintenance treatment is essential to the well-being of bipolar patients. Although mood stabilization tends to be the immediate goal of psychopharmacologic intervention, clinicians should also consider potential suicidality when treating a bipolar patient. Appropriate maintenance treatment can substantially reduce the risk of suicide (Baethge et al. 2003; Coppen and Farmer 1998; Tondo and Baldessarini 2000, 2001a), but how do we decide what constitutes "appropriate maintenance" when it comes to suicide prevention? Although a variety of mood stabilizers, antidepressants, and antipsychotics have been the focus of research in this realm, the answer is not eminently clear.

Lithium

Given its frequent and historical use in bipolar illness, it is not surprising that lithium has received a great deal of attention in research concerning psychopharmacology and suicide prevention in patients with mood disorders. A variety of meta-analyses, smaller independent studies, and study of lithium and anticonvulsants in two large health insurance databases generally substantiate a cautiously optimistic view of lithium as a prophylactic agent against suicide in bipolar disorder. While research on lithium's protective effects is promising, it is also essential to keep in mind the complications surrounding the research designs as well as the daily clinical problems of treatment noncompliance in the bipolar population.

Goodwin et al. (2004) reported a strong effect favoring lithium compared with divalproex sodium in 20,638 members of two large health maintenance organizations in the United States. The incidence of emergency department admissions for suicide attempts (31.3 for valproate vs. 10.8 for lithium per 1,000 persons/year), suicide attempts resulting in hospitalization (10.5 vs. 4.2 per 1,000 persons/year), and suicidal death (1.7 vs. 0.7 per 1,000 persons/year) were all lower in lithium-treated patients. After adjustment for a number of demographic factors, including age and psychiatric and medical comorbidity, the risk of suicide death was reported to be 2.7 times greater for patients prescribed divalproex for a diagnosis of bipolar disorder compared to those prescribed lithium. Although intriguing, the nonrandomized nature of the sample leaves open the concern that the groups were clinically different. For instance, it is not known how many of the patients in the divalproex group had previously failed to respond to lithium and were thus a treatment-resistant group. In any case, the results are strongly in favor of lithium and are consistent with other examinations of the effect of lithium on suicidality.

A case-control study by Modestin and Schwarzenbach (1992) found that matched controls discharged within 1 year from an inpatient psychiatric hospitalization were more likely to be on lithium than those who committed suicide, yet were equally likely to have dropped out of treatment. Whether this represents a protective effect from lithium is unclear.

A meta-analysis of 33 studies investigating long-term lithium treatment between 1970 and 2000 yields results that overwhelmingly favor lithium as a potential means of suicide prevention (Baldessarini et al. 2001). Of the 19 studies comparing groups with and without lithium treatment, 18 found a lower risk of suicide in the treatment group and one had no suicides in either group. The results clearly present a favorable association of lithium with decreased suicidality. Overall, the meta-analysis demonstrates a thirteenfold reduction in suicidality for patients with an affective illness, leading to a largely reduced risk, which nevertheless remains larger than that estimated for the general population. Specifically, the rates of suicide associated with lithium treatment (0.109%–0.224% annually) are 10 times greater than the international base rate (0.017%) (Baldessarini et al. 2001). Thus, in spite of the prophylaxis afforded by lithium against suicidality, its protective effects appear to be somewhat incomplete.

A second meta-analysis concerning lithium use in bipolar disorder further supports the claim of a demonstrably decreased suicide risk in patients treated with lithium. Tondo and Baldessarini's (2000) review of 22 studies reveals a sevenfold decrease in suicides for patients treated with lithium as compared to those not receiving lithium or having discontinued it. The suicide rate for the group receiving lithium treatment was approximately 0.227% per year, while the group without lithium treatment was 1.778±1.444% per year. As with the meta-analysis discussed above, however, the decreased rates associated with lithium treatment are still significantly greater than those found in the general population; in this case, by 13.7 times. In spite of the high risk (compared with the normal population) of suicide in the group treated with lithium, it appears that the risk of suicide attempts is decreased to a greater extent with lithium treatment. In fact, the rate of suicide attempts associated with lithium treatment may actually be less than the rate of suicide attempts in the general population (0.255% annually vs. 0.315% annually).

A third meta-analysis of 32 randomized, controlled trials was recently reported (Cipriani et al. 2005). In these studies, 1,389 patients were randomized to lithium and 2,069 to other agents, including placebo (n=779), antidepressants (n=247), and other mood stabilizers and combination treatments. Lithium treatment was associated with a reduced likelihood to die by suicide (2 vs. 11 suicides, odds ratio=0.26, 95% confidence interval [CI]=0.09–0.77), a reduced likelihood for self-injurious behavior (0 vs. 7 events, odds 0.21, 95% CI=0.08–0.50), and reduced death from any reason (9 vs. 22, odds ratio = 0.42, 95% CI=0.21–0.87). It follows that lithium may exert particularly strong protective effects for patients who are less inclined to commit suicidal acts with the intention of suicide completion. In other words, although lithium may not lower suicide rates in patients with mood disorders to the level found in the general population, the fact that it seems to drastically reduce the frequency of attempts demonstrates its protective properties.

Several notes must be made regarding the reliability of these meta-analyses, given several substantial limitations. First, the majority of the studies reviewed in both did not seek to address suicidality as a primary outcome variable (Baldessarini et al. 2001; Tondo and Baldessarini 2000). Second, it is noteworthy that the results of these meta-analyses were likely tainted by the presence of a variety of diagnoses in the study samples. Frequent inclusion of individuals with diagnoses of major depressive disorder and schizoaffective disorder confounds our understanding of the effects of lithium in a strictly bipolar population. Additionally, given the high rates of comorbidity in affective illness (i.e., whether the secondary or tertiary diagnosis is one of substance abuse, an anxiety disorder, an Axis II disorder, etc.), it would be instructive to parse out the effects of lithium for patients with a comorbid illness and those with a "pure" bipolar diagnosis. Furthermore, lithium has historically been the first-line treatment; severely ill patients or lithium nonresponders may have disproportionally higher suicide rates. Fortunately, several individual studies address these limitations and may present us with a fuller illustration of lithium effects in specific segments of the bipolar spectrum.

It is difficult to confidently generalize results of many psychopharmacologic studies to the general bipolar population involving lithium because of the lack of trials applying a randomized design. Tondo, Hennen, and Baldessarini's (2001b) meta-analysis indicated that among 22 studies comparing a group with lithium treatment with a group without this treatment, only three were double-blind, randomized, controlled trials (RCTs). However, these trials further substantiate and strengthen the claim that lithium exerts a protective effect against suicide. In fact, in 328 patients not receiving lithium therapy and 369 receiving lithium (yielded by an analyses of the three RCTs mentioned above), 1.28% per year committed suicide in the former group compared with 0.00% per year in the latter. An additional analysis of nine RCTs involving lithium found similar rates and further illustrates lithium's protective effects against suicide (Burgess 2002; Tondo et al. 2001b). Notably, no study found a negative effect for lithium, and although not all of the studies found statistically significant effects, all effects were in the same direction (i.e., lithium was associated with a lower suicide rate). Given the prospective and randomized designs of these studies, they provide strong support for the use of lithium in patients with mood disorders judged to be at risk for suicidal behavior.

Reasonable rates of treatment compliance are necessary if we are to expect psychopharmacologic interventions to exert the desired effects, yet treatment compliance is a constant struggle for many bipolar patients. In issues of suicidality, particularly with respect to a medication with promising protective effects, compliance may be especially worthy of attention. In fact, it appears that compliance with lithium treatment may not only decrease the risk of suicide but that it may actually decrease general mortality rates. In a sample of 103 patients treated with lithium and followed over the course of 11 years, the projected number of deaths was 18.31 (based on demographic factors for the population), while the actual number of deaths was 10 (Coppen et al. 1991), with no suicides. The authors concluded that lithium may compensate for the high mortality rate found in mood disorders and actually reverse it. Notably, the study sample was highly treatment compliant, with only 10 patients discontinuing treatment over the course of study duration. Alternately, Brodersen et al. (2000) found that over the course of 16 years of observation, 40 of the 133 study participants who were treated with lithium died, with 11 deaths resulting from suicide. While these results could be taken as further support for the theory that lithium possesses an incomplete protective effect, further examination of the study sample indicates that treatment noncompliance may have been a strong risk factor for death. In fact, individuals who were not compliant with their lithium treatment were four times more likely to die from suicide than those who were compliant, although these findings were marginally insignificant ($P=0.06$). Direct conclusions as to the direction of causality in such a study are impossible. Perhaps lithium does not have as strong a protective effect as is believed or perhaps its negative side effects lead to higher rates of noncompliance. Regardless of the reason, noncompliance is a serious problem in bipolar patients and must be addressed if we are to expect that lithium will provide prophylaxis against suicidality.

The potential dangers associated with lithium discontinuation may further inform our understanding of lithium's effects on suicidality. It appears that rapid or accelerated lithium discontinuation (as may be practiced by noncompliant individuals who decide to simply stop taking their medications) places a person at serious risk for suicidal behavior. In a sample of 165 patients who decided to discontinue lithium for a variety of reasons (whether electively or for some medical reason), the rate of all suicidal acts rose 14 times following discontinuation (Tondo and Baldessarini 2000). In another sample of 128 individuals who chose to discontinue lithium, the rate of suicide-related deaths rose to 1.27% per year from 0.101% per year with lithium maintenance treatment (Baldessarini et al. 1999). Overall mortality in a group of 273 subjects followed after lithium discontinuation was much higher than in the general population, with a standardized mortality ratio (SMR) of 2.5 for the discontinuation group (the SMR for the general population was 1.0). The authors concluded that this is higher than the SMR for patients continued on lithium in their other data, but because there is no direct comparison, it is not possible to estimate the actual effect of lithium discontinuation on mortality (Muller-Oerlinghausen et al. 1996).

It is unclear whether the risk of suicide following lithium discontinuation exceeds that found in untreated affective illness. However, the striking increase in suicides following lithium discontinuation demonstrates the need for vigilance and frequent communication with patients at risk for suicidal actions. Effective management of adverse side effects or other reasons for which patients may choose to discontinue lithium treatment is also warranted. The effects of lithium discontinuation speak further to the benefits of long-term lithium maintenance therapy. Lithium discontinuation can also contribute to suicidality indirectly; some have suggested that it may lead to higher relapse rates and a refractory response to future lithium treatment (Post et al. 1992).

Several theories have been proposed regarding the mechanisms of suicide prevention afforded by lithium. It is possible that decreased suicidality is simply one of the additional benefits accompanying the mood stabilization afforded by lithium. However, it also seems probable that lithium has additional protective properties. Serotonin mediation may be a primary means through which lithium exerts these effects. Specifically, lithium's actions in the forebrain may address the potential serotonergic deficiencies that are associated with self-harm and violence (Mann et al. 1999a, 1999b). These effects are not associated with the mood-stabilizing properties of carbamazepine and may explain why lithium has been found to be superior to carbamazepine in suicide prevention (Greil et al. 1997).

Lithium may be the first-line choice for clinical management of suicide risk; however, it is essential that study results be interpreted and clinically applied with caution and careful consideration. Ultimately, although the effects of lithium are promising in the realm of suicide prevention, they have not yet been definitively determined. A greater variety of RCTs specifically designed to measure the anti-suicide effects of lithium are needed for a better understanding of this relationship. Additionally, it is essential that we not neglect the potential protective effects of other psychiatric medications aside from lithium, particularly as an option for lithium nonresponders and patients who cannot tolerate lithium. These individuals may be at a higher risk of suicide attempts and completion (Muller-Oerlinghausen et al. 1992).

Anticonvulsants

There are almost no data available to judge whether any anticonvulsants typically used in the treatment of bipolar disorder have a prophylactic effect against suicidality. Lamotrigine and divalproex are two anticonvulsants that have been studied in the maintenance treatment of bipolar disorder and that may have some prophylactic efficacy in the prevention of depressive episodes. The evidence that lamotrigine prevents episodes of depressive relapse is particularly robust, but the drug is only recently becoming widely used, and there have been no longitudinal trials examining the question of suicide prevention with it (Goodwin et al. 2004). Divalproex may have some prophylactic effect against the return of depression, but no adequate data exist to support its use for that purpose (Gyulai et al. 2003). Despite its flaws, the Goodwin et al. (2003) study concluded that lithium was superior to divalproex for the prevention of hospitalization for suicidal ideation and suicide attempts, yet it was not designed to determine whether divalproex was superior to other treatments for bipolar disorder in suicide prevention.

In a randomized, maintenance trial of bipolar disorder, 171 patients received either lithium or carbamazepine and were followed for 2.5 years (Kleindienst and Greil 2000). Although there were no suicides during this time, four subjects taking carbamazepine made suicide attempts whereas none of the subjects on lithium did. This difference was not significant, but it was consistent with the data suggesting that lithium prevents suicide.

Atypical Antipsychotics

Atypical antipsychotics are increasingly used as first-line treatment for bipolar disorder, in both acute mania and acute depression as well as in maintenance treatment. Because of the increased use of antipsychotics and their potential replacement of lithium and anticonvulsants (such as valproate), in clinical decision-making with patients, their utility in preventing suicide should be explored. The strongest data suggesting a suicide preventive effect of atypical antipsychotics come from the international suicide prevention trial (interSePT), which found that the risk of suicide in schizophrenia was significantly decreased with clozapine versus olanzapine (Meltzer et al. 2003). This study, however, did not include patients with bipolar disorder, and its generalizability to mood disorders is uncertain.

There are some suggestions that atypical antipsychotics may have some anti-suicide potential in bipolar disorder. In a post hoc analysis of a trial of olanzapine added to lithium or divalproex for mixed or manic episodes, suicidality ratings dropped significantly for patients with dysphoric mania who were given olanzapine. Total 21-item Hamilton Rating Scale for Depression scores were also significantly decreased (Baker et al. 2004). However, because this study was not designed to address the potential of olanzapine to prevent suicidality, it remains unclear how meaningful the results are.

Antidepressants

As commonly used as antidepressants are in the treatment of bipolar disorder, their utility in the treatment of bipolar depression remains unclear (Altshuler et al. 2003; Ghaemi et al. 2004; Nemeroff et al. 2001). There are no data to suggest whether they are of utility in preventing suicide. In a study of 78 patients with unipolar or bipolar disorder treated with antidepressants, bipolar patients were more likely to switch to mania, develop rapid cycling, and lose antidepressant response (Ghaemi et al. 2004). Although the study is limited by its retrospective design, it does suggest that, for some patients, risk factors for suicide might increase during antidepressant treatment.

A recent report by Jick et al. (2004) suggests that the risk for suicidal behavior increases in the first month after the initiation of antidepressant treatment—especially in the first nine days. Muller-Oerlinghausen and Berghofer (1999) have suggested that SSRI antidepressants may increase suicidal thoughts through akathesia or by energizing depressed patients, but the risk for this (especially in bipolar disorder) is unknown. In their review, they concluded that while lithium may have anti-suicide potential, this effect has not been shown for antidepressants or for nonlithium mood stabilizers.

In a population study in England, Morgan et al. (2004) found that the increase in antidepressant prescriptions between 1993 and 2002 was associated with decreased suicide rates, which fell from 98.2 to 84.3 per million population. Although they could not draw a causal relationship between antidepressant use and suicide reduction, they suggested that the more widespread use of less lethal antidepressants than of tricyclic antidepressants may contribute to this. Whether this association would remain in the subset of the population with bipolar disorder is unknown.

Psychotherapy

There are no studies that suggest or confirm the utility of specific psychotherapies in the prevention of suicide in bipolar disorder. Rucci et al. (2002) made the most ambitious attempt to do so. Between 1991 and 2000, 175 subjects with bipolar I disorder or schizoaffective manic disorder were followed. All were stabilized for at least 4 weeks on lithium and randomly assigned to receive social rhythm therapy or intensive clinical management. The suicide rate, which had been 1.05 per 100 persons/month before the trial, decreased by two-thirds during the study. While no differences between the two groups could be found, the authors concluded that comprehensive treatment, including psychosocial treatment, might be effective in preventing suicide in this population (Rucci et al. 2002). It is unclear whether this decreased risk was due to the efficacy of the lithium treatment (all the patients, by definition, were lithium responsive), although there is an argument to be made that combined treatment contributed to the effect.

Therapies that target and ameliorate the psychosocial risk factors associated with increased suicide in bipolar disorder may have some suicide preventive effect, as suggested by Gray and Otto (2001). They reviewed 17 randomized studies of psychotherapy for bipolar disorder and concluded that therapies that are successful at enabling patients to easily elicit emergency care through simple interventions—those that increase social problem-solving skills and those that combine problem-solving with cognitive, social, emotional labeling, and distress-tolerance skills—would likely have the biggest effect. The authors pointed out that the therapies that have shown some efficacy in symptom reduction and relapse prevention in bipolar disorder—family-focused treatment (FFT), interpersonal therapy with a social rhythm component (IPSRT), and cognitive-behavioral therapy (CBT)—have not yet shown efficacy in reducing suicide. These therapies may prove useful yet as they all have a problem-solving component. CBT, for instance, has shown utility in reducing depression and hopelessness in unipolar depression and may do so for bipolar depression; if this is the case, a major risk factor for depression may be decreased by this treatment.

SUICIDE PREDICTION

There are characteristics that are overrepresented in bipolar patients with suicidality (Table 5–1): hopelessness, aggressivity, severity of depressed mood, and suicidal ideation have been repeatedly found to be associated with suicidality (Ahrens and Linden 1996; Beck et al. 1993; Brown et al. 2000; Minkoff et al. 1973; Oquendo and Mann 2001). These symptoms are neither specific to bipolar disorder, nor easily accounted for by any component of the clinical presentation of the patient with bipolar disorder. A complex matrix of mood disorder, family history and genetics, comorbidity (especially anxiety and substance use, including nicotine), medical history (including head injury), and social and economic factors may contribute to the presence and severity of these symptoms. While not all are amenable to clinical intervention, many are, and awareness by the clinician and the social network of the bipolar patient may contribute to reducing risk and increasing the probability of suicide prevention.

Mann and Oquendo have proposed a stress diathesis model of suicide in bipolar disorder, in which aggressive or suicidal behavior is influenced by a cascade of factors (Mann et al. 1999b; Oquendo and Mann 2001). The interaction of mood disorder and social factors leads to hopelessness, impulsivity, and suicidal ideation, in part influenced by trait factors (such as serotonin functioning), decreased cognitive functioning due to head injury, and substance use (including drugs, alcohol, and nicotine). Mann et al. (1999b) suggests that the monitoring of these separate factors should be a part of ongoing suicide prevention in bipolar disorder.

Accurate suicide prediction, however, is nearly impossible. As Sachs et al. (2001) have explained, the positive predictive value—the true positives for an outcome divided by the total positives (true positives plus

TABLE 5–1. Prominent risk factors for suicide in bipolar disorder

- Past suicide attempt
- Early age at onset (<18 years)
- Early in course of illness
- Period immediately after hospital admission
- Period immediately after hospital discharge
- Recurrent depressive episodes (>4)
- Adult or childhood sexual abuse
- Social isolation
- Nicotine dependence
- Other substance or alcohol dependence
- Comorbid anxiety disorder
- Cluster B personality disorder
- Hopelessness
- Impulsivity
- Depression
- Mixed state or mania with significant depressive symptoms
- Suicidal ideation

false positives)—of suicide assessment is extremely low. They proposed that a model for suicide prevention should include an assessment of factors that may increase inclination for suicide (e.g., suicidal ideation and hopelessness) on a matrix with an assessment of the opportunity for making a suicide attempt (e.g., owning a weapon, having a large stock of pills, being alone). Inclination and opportunity can each be estimated as high, moderate, or low, and the intervention can be tailored to the estimated risk. The lowest risk would merit a treatment plan to manage the development of suicidal ideation, along with preventative psychopharmacologic management, such as lithium. The highest risk would merit an emergency intervention, such as hospitalization, but may include the mobilization of social supports, the removal of the means for suicide, and acute treatment for depression. The goal for management is to match intervention to need.

Clinicians should first use treatments in bipolar disorder that have sound scientific underpinnings. For high-risk patients, a trial of lithium and ongoing management with it may be the intervention with the greatest likelihood of success. The reduction of depression and depressive recurrence should be a hallmark of care, and until the anti-suicide effects of a specific treatment can be established in larger trials, the treatment approach should be based on current research.

Although they are not proven to prevent suicide, interventions targeting comorbid conditions may decrease the theoretical risk of it. Anxiety disorders should be adequately treated, both with pharmacological interventions and with psychotherapy effective for the specific disorder. The use of antidepressants to treat anxiety should be undertaken cautiously, but prominent anxiety symptoms should be minimized as much as possible. Interventions to reduce substance use are rarely used in bipolar disorder, but clinicians should be prepared to access them, both in terms of psychopharmacology (e.g., buprenorphine for opiate dependence, acamprosate for alcohol dependence) and psychosocial treatments.

One of the most prominent comorbidities in bipolar disorder, nicotine dependence, is a most powerful predictor of suicide. Although no interventions for smoking cessation have been validated in bipolar disorder and the impact of quitting smoking on suicide risk is unknown, it may nevertheless be of great benefit to the patient to stop smoking. Current standard treatments for smoking cessation are likely safe, if not effective, in bipolar disorder.

SUMMARY

While suicide itself is a rare event, the prevention of suicide must be a consistent and ongoing effort between treaters, patients, and patients' families and social networks. A patient is never completely safe from suicide risk, and assessment of suicide must be a part of each clinical encounter. While most suicides occur early in the illness, the risk remains elevated over the lifetime of the patient. With patients who have ongoing recovery from mood episodes, it may not be necessary to make suicide assessment a centerpiece of every visit, although information about it must be sought—whether through patient self-report forms or through direct verbal inquiry—at each encounter. Suicide assessment must be undertaken during both acute and maintenance treatment, and interventions appropriate to the patient's symptoms and history must be offered.

REFERENCES

Ahrens B, Linden M: Is there a suicidality syndrome independent of specific major psychiatric disorder? Results of a split half multiple regression analysis. Acta Psychiatr Scand 94:79–86, 1996

Altshuler L, Suppes T, Black D, et al: Impact of antidepressant discontinuation after acute bipolar depression remission on rates of depressive relapse at 1-year follow-up. Am J Psychiatry 160:1252–1262, 2003

Angst J, Preisig M: Outcome of a clinical cohort of unipolar, bipolar and schizoaffective patients. Results of a prospective study from 1959 to 1985. Schweiz Arch Neurol Psychiatr 146:17–23, 1995

Angst J, Gerber-Werder R, Zuberbuhler HU, et al: Is bipolar I disorder heterogeneous? Eur Arch Psychiatry Clin Neurosci 254:82–91, 2004

Baethge C, Gruschka P, Smolka MN, et al: Effectiveness and outcome predictors of long-term lithium prophylaxis in unipolar major depressive disorder. J Psychiatry Neurosci 28:355–361, 2003

Baker RW, Brown E, Akiskal HS, et al: Efficacy of olanzapine combined with valproate or lithium in the treatment of dysphoric mania. Br J Psychiatry 185:472–478, 2004

Baldessarini RJ, Tondo L, Hennen J: Effects of lithium treatment and its discontinuation on suicide behavior in bipolar manic depressive disorders. J Clin Psychiatry 60 (suppl 2):77–84, 1999

Baldessarini RJ, Tondo L, Hennen J: Treating the suicidal patient with bipolar disorder. Reducing suicide risk with lithium. Ann N Y Acad Sci 932:24–38, 2001

Beck AT, Steer RA, Brown G: Dysfunctional attitudes and suicidal ideation in psychiatric outpatients. Suicide Life Threat Behav 23:11–20, 1993

Berglund M, Nilsson K: Mortality in severe depression. A prospective study including 103 suicides. Acta Psychiatr Scand 76:372–380, 1987

Blair-West GW, Mellsop GW, Eyeson-Annan ML: Down-rating lifetime suicide risk in major depression. Acta Psychiatr Scand 95:259–263, 1997

Bocchetta A, Chillotti C, Carboni G, et al: Association of personal and familial suicide risk with low serum cholesterol concentration in male lithium patients. Acta Psychiatr Scand 104:37–41, 2001

Bonnier B, Gorwood P, Hamon M, et al: Association of 5-HT$_{(2A)}$ receptor gene polymorphism with major affective disorders: the case of a subgroup of bipolar disorder with low suicide risk. Biol Psychiatry 51:762–765, 2002

Bostwick JM, Pankratz VS: Affective disorders and suicide risk: a reexamination. Am J Psychiatry 157:1925–1932, 2000

Brieger P, Ehrt U, Marneros A: Frequency of comorbid personality disorders in bipolar and unipolar affective disorders. Compr Psychiatry 44:28–34, 2003

Brodersen A, Licht RW, Vestergaard P, et al: Sixteen-year mortality in patients with affective disorder commenced on lithium. Br J Psychiatry 176:429–433, 2000

Brodsky BS, Malone KM, Ellis SP, et al: Characteristics of borderline personality disorder associated with suicidal behavior. Am J Psychiatry 154:1715–1719, 1997

Brown GK, Beck AT, Steer RA, et al: Risk factors for suicide in psychiatric outpatients: a 20-year prospective study. J Consult Clin Psychol 68:371–377, 2000

Carter TD, Mundo E, Parikh SV, et al: Early age at onset as a risk factor for poor outcome of bipolar disorder. J Psychiatr Res 37:297–303, 2003

Cassidy F, Carroll BJ: Frequencies of signs and symptoms in mixed and pure episodes of mania: implications for the study of manic episodes. Prog Neuropsychopharmacol Biol Psychiatry 25:659–665, 2001

Chen YW, Dilsaver SC: Lifetime rates of suicide attempts among subjects with bipolar and unipolar disorders relative to subjects with other Axis I disorders. Biol Psychiatry 39:896–899, 1996

Coppen A, Farmer R: Suicide mortality in patients on lithium maintenance therapy. J Affect Disord 50:261–267, 1998

Coppen A, Standish-Barry H, Bailey J, et al: Does lithium reduce the mortality of recurrent mood disorders? J Affect Disord 23:1–7, 1991

Corcos M, Taieb O, Benoit-Lamy S, et al: Suicide attempts in women with bulimia nervosa: frequency and characteristics. Acta Psychiatr Scand 106:381–386, 2002

Coryell W, Solomon D, Turvey C, et al: The long-term course of rapid-cycling bipolar disorder. Arch Gen Psychiatry 60:914–920, 2003

Dalton EJ, Cate-Carter TD, Mundo E, et al: Suicide risk in bipolar patients: the role of co-morbid substance use disorders. Bipolar Disord 5:58–61, 2003

Dilsaver SC, Chen YW, Swann AC, et al: Suicidality in patients with pure and depressive mania. Am J Psychiatry 151:1312–1315, 1994

Fagiolini A, Kupfer DJ, Rucci P, et al: Suicide attempts and ideation in patients with bipolar I disorder. J Clin Psychiatry 65:509–514, 2004

Feinman JA, Dunner DL: The effect of alcohol and substance abuse on the course of bipolar affective disorder. J Affect Disord 37:43–49, 1996

Frank E, Cyranowski JM, Rucci P, et al: Clinical significance of lifetime panic spectrum symptoms in the treatment of patients with bipolar I disorder. Arch Gen Psychiatry 59:905–911, 2002

Ghaemi SN, Rosenquist KJ, Ko JY, et al: Antidepressant treatment in bipolar versus unipolar depression. Am J Psychiatry 161:163–165, 2004

Goodwin FK, Jamison KR: Manic-Depressive Illness. New York, Oxford University Press, 1990

Goodwin FK, Fireman B, Simon GE, et al: Suicide risk in bipolar disorder during treatment with lithium and divalproex. JAMA 290:1467–1473, 2003

Goodwin GM, Bowden CL, Calabrese JR, et al: A pooled analysis of 2 placebo-controlled 18-month trials of lamotrigine and lithium maintenance in bipolar I disorder. J Clin Psychiatry 65:432–441, 2004

Gray SM, Otto MW: Psychosocial approaches to suicide prevention: applications to patients with bipolar disorder. J Clin Psychiatry 62 (suppl 25):56–64, 2001

Greil W, Ludwig-Mayerhofer W, Erazo N, et al: Lithium versus carbamazepine in the maintenance treatment of bipolar disorders—a randomised study. J Affect Disord 43:151–161, 1997

Grunebaum MF, Oquendo MA, Harkavy-Friedman JM, et al: Delusions and suicidality. Am J Psychiatry 158:742–747, 2001

Guze SB, Robins E: Suicide and primary affective disorders. Br J Psychiatry 117:437–438, 1970

Gyulai L, Bowden CL, McElroy SL, et al: Maintenance efficacy of divalproex in the prevention of bipolar depression. Neuropsychopharmacology 28:1374–1382, 2003

Henry C, Van den Bulke D, Bellivier F, et al: Anxiety disorders in 318 bipolar patients: prevalence and impact on illness severity and response to mood stabilizer. J Clin Psychiatry 64:331–335, 2003

Hoyer EH, Olesen AV, Mortensen PB: Suicide risk in patients hospitalised because of an affective disorder: a follow-up study, 1973–1993. J Affect Disord 78:209–217, 2004

Inskip HM, Harris EC, Barraclough B: Lifetime risk of suicide for affective disorder, alcoholism, and schizophrenia. Br J Psychiatry 172:35–37, 1998

Isometsa ET, Henriksson MM, Aro HM, et al: Suicide in bipolar disorder in Finland. Am J Psychiatry 151:1020–1024, 1994

Jick H, Kaye JA, Jick SS: Antidepressants and the risk of suicidal behaviors. JAMA 292:338–343, 2004

Judd LL, Akiskal HS, Schettler PJ, et al: The long-term natural history of the weekly symptomatic status of bipolar I disorder. Arch Gen Psychiatry 59:530–537, 2002

Judd LL, Akiskal HS, Schettler PJ, et al: A prospective investigation of the natural history of the long-term weekly symptomatic status of bipolar II disorder. Arch Gen Psychiatry 60:261–269, 2003

Kelly TM, Cornelius JR, Lynch KG: Psychiatric and substance use disorders as risk factors for attempted suicide among adolescents: a case control study. Suicide Life Threat Behav 32:301–312, 2002

Kessler RC, McGonagle KA, Zao S, et al: Lifetime and 12-month prevalence of DSM-III-R psychiatric disorders in the United States. Results from the National Comorbidity Survey. Arch Gen Psychiatry 51:8–19, 1994

Kessler RC, Chiu WT, Demler O, et al: Prevalence, severity, and comorbidity of 12-month DSM-IV disorders in the National Comorbidity Survey Replication. Arch Gen Psychiatry 62:617–627, 2005; erratum 62:709, 2005

Kleindienst N, Greil W: Differential efficacy of lithium and carbamazepine in the prophylaxis of bipolar disorder: results of the MAP study. Neuropsychobiology 42 (suppl 1):2–10, 2000

Krishnan KR: Psychiatric and medical comorbidities of bipolar disorder. Psychosom Med 67:1–8, 2005

Leverich GS, Altshuler LL, Frye MA, et al: Factors associated with suicide attempts in 648 patients with bipolar disorder in the Stanley Foundation Bipolar Network. J Clin Psychiatry 64:506–515, 2003

Levine J, Chengappa KN, Brar JS, et al: Illness characteristics and their association with prescription patterns for bipolar I disorder. Bipolar Disord 3:41–49, 2001

MacKinnon DF, Zandi PP, Gershon E, et al: Rapid switching of mood in families with multiple cases of bipolar disorder. Arch Gen Psychiatry 60:921–928, 2003

Malone KM, Waternaux C, Haas GL, et al: Cigarette smoking, suicidal behavior, and serotonin function in major psychiatric disorders. Am J Psychiatry 160:773–779, 2003

Mann JJ, Oquendo M, Underwood MD, et al: The neurobiology of suicide risk: a review for the clinician. J Clin Psychiatry 60 (suppl 2):7–11; 1999; discussion 60 (suppl 2):18–20, 113–116, 1999a

Mann JJ, Waternaux C, Haas GL, et al: Toward a clinical model of suicidal behavior in psychiatric patients. Am J Psychiatry 156:181–189, 1999b

Massat I, Souery D, Lipp O, et al: A European multicenter association study of 5-HTR2A receptor polymorphism in bipolar affective disorder. Am J Med Genet 96:136–140, 2000

McElroy SL, Altshuler LL, Suppes T, et al: Axis I psychiatric comorbidity and its relationship to historical illness variables in 288 patients with bipolar disorder. Am J Psychiatry 158:420–426, 2001

Meltzer HY, Alphs L, Green AI, et al: Clozapine treatment for suicidality in schizophrenia: International Suicide Prevention Trial (InterSePT). Arch Gen Psychiatry 60:82–91, 2003; erratum 60:735, 2003

Minkoff K, Bergman E, Beck AT, et al: Hopelessness, depression, and attempted suicide. Am J Psychiatry 130:455–459, 1973

Modestin J, Schwarzenbach F: Effect of psychopharmacotherapy on suicide risk in discharged psychiatric inpatients. Acta Psychiatr Scand 85:173–175, 1992

Moffitt TE, Brammer GL, Caspi A, et al: Whole blood serotonin relates to violence in an epidemiological study. Biol Psychiatry 43:446–457, 1998

Morgan OW, Griffiths C, Majeed A: Association between mortality from suicide in England and antidepressant prescribing: an ecological study. BMC Public Health 4:63, 2004

Morrison JR: Bipolar affective disorder and alcoholism. Am J Psychiatry 131:1130–1133, 1974

Muller-Oerlinghausen B, Berghofer A: Antidepressants and suicidal risk. J Clin Psychiatry 60 (suppl 2):94–99, 1999; discussion 60 (suppl 2):111–116, 1999

Muller-Oerlinghausen B, Ahrens B, Grof E, et al: The effect of long-term lithium treatment on the mortality of patients with manic-depressive and schizoaffective illness. Acta Psychiatr Scand 86:218–222, 1992

Muller-Oerlinghausen B, Wolf T, Ahrens B, et al: Mortality of patients who dropped out from regular lithium prophylaxis: a collaborative study by the International Group for the Study of Lithium-treated patients (IGSLI). Acta Psychiatr Scand 94:344–347, 1996

Nemeroff CB, Evans DL, Gyulai L, et al: Double-blind, placebo-controlled comparison of imipramine and paroxetine in the treatment of bipolar depression. Am J Psychiatry 158:906–912, 2001

Ni X, Trakalo JM, Mundo E, et al: Family based association study of the serotonin-2A receptor gene (5-HT$_{2A}$) and bipolar disorder. Neuromolecular Med 2:251–259, 2002

Oquendo MA, Mann JJ: Identifying and managing suicide risk in bipolar patients. J Clin Psychiatry 62 (suppl 25):31–34, 2001

Oquendo MA, Placidi GP, Malone KM, et al: Positron emission tomography of regional brain metabolic responses to a serotonergic challenge and lethality of suicide attempts in major depression. Arch Gen Psychiatry 60:14–22, 2003

Oquendo MA, Galfalvy H, Russo S, et al: Prospective study of clinical predictors of suicidal acts after a major depressive episode in patients with major depressive disorder or bipolar disorder. Am J Psychiatry 161:1433–1441, 2004

Perlis RH, Miyahara S, Marangell LB, et al: Long-term implications of early onset in bipolar disorder: data from the first 1000 participants in the systematic treatment enhancement program for bipolar disorder (STEP-BD). Biol Psychiatry 55:875–881, 2004

Post RM, Leverich GS, Altshuler L, et al: Lithium-discontinuation-induced refractoriness: preliminary observations. Am J Psychiatry 149:1727–1729, 1992

Raja M, Azzoni A: Suicide attempts: differences between unipolar and bipolar patients and among groups with different lethality risk. J Affect Disord 82:437–442, 2004

Regier DA, Farmer ME, Rae DS, et al: Comorbidity of mental disorders with alcohol and other drug abuse: results from the Epidemiologic Catchment Area (ECA) Study. JAMA 264:2511–2518, 1990

Roy-Byrne PP, Post RM, Hambrick DD, et al: Suicide and course of illness in major affective disorder. J Affect Disord 15:1–8, 1988

Rucci P, Frank E, Kostelnik B, et al: Suicide attempts in patients with bipolar I disorder during acute and maintenance phases of intensive treatment with pharmacotherapy and adjunctive psychotherapy. Am J Psychiatry 159:1160–1164, 2002

Sachs GS, Yan LJ, Swann AC, et al: Integration of suicide prevention into outpatient management of bipolar disorder. J Clin Psychiatry 62 (suppl 25):3–11, 2001

Simon NM, Otto MW, Weiss RD, et al: Pharmacotherapy for bipolar disorder and comorbid conditions: baseline data from STEP-BD. J Clin Psychopharmacol 24:512–520, 2004

Simpson SG, Jamison KR: The risk of suicide in patients with bipolar disorders. J Clin Psychiatry 60 (suppl 2):53–56, 1999

Slama F, Bellivier F, Henry C, et al: Bipolar patients with suicidal behavior: toward the identification of a clinical subgroup. J Clin Psychiatry 65:1035–1039, 2004

Stein D, Lilenfeld LR, Wildman PC, et al: Attempted suicide and self-injury in patients diagnosed with eating disorders. Compr Psychiatry 45:447–451, 2004

Strakowski SM, Tohen M, Stoll AL, et al: Comorbidity in mania at first hospitalization. Am J Psychiatry 149:554–556, 1992

Strakowski SM, McElroy SL, Keck PE Jr, et al: Suicidality among patients with mixed and manic bipolar disorder. Am J Psychiatry 153:674–676, 1996

Tondo L, Baldessarini RJ: Reduced suicide risk during lithium maintenance treatment. J Clin Psychiatry 61 (suppl 9):97–104, 2000

Tondo L, Baldessarini RJ, Hennen J, et al: Suicide attempts in major affective disorder patients with comorbid substance use disorders. J Clin Psychiatry 60 (suppl 2):63–69, 1999; discussion 60 (suppl 2):75–76, 113–116, 1999

Tondo L, Ghiani C, Albert M: Pharmacologic interventions in suicide prevention. J Clin Psychiatry 62 (suppl 25):51–55, 2001a

Tondo L, Hennen J, Baldessarini RJ: Lower suicide risk with long-term lithium treatment in major affective illness: a meta-analysis. Acta Psychiatr Scand 104:163–172, 2001b

Tsai SY, Kuo CJ, Chen CC, et al: Risk factors for completed suicide in bipolar disorder. J Clin Psychiatry 63:469–476, 2002

Tut TG, Wang JL, Lim CC: Negative association between T102C polymorphism at the 5-HT2A receptor gene and bipolar affective disorders in Singaporean Chinese. J Affect Disord 58:211–214, 2000

Vieta E, Colom F, Martinez-Aran A, et al: Bipolar II disorder and comorbidity. Compr Psychiatry 41:339–343, 2000

Wu LH, Dunner DL: Suicide attempts in rapid cycling bipolar disorder patients. J Affect Disord 29:57–61, 1993

Zureik M, Courbon D, Ducimetière P: Serum cholesterol concentration and death from suicide in men: Paris prospective study I. Br Med J 313:649–651, 1996

TREATMENT AND PREVENTION OF BIPOLAR DEPRESSION

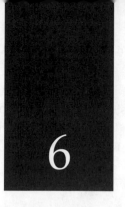

6

LITHIUM AND ANTIEPILEPTIC DRUGS IN BIPOLAR DEPRESSION

Rif S. El-Mallakh, M.D.

LITHIUM HAS BEEN THE GOLD STANDARD for the treatment of bipolar illness for over 50 years (Schou 2001). There is more clinical and research experience with this drug than any other used to treat bipolar illness. Its utility in depression has been demonstrated in older studies and is generally underappreciated by the current generation of psychiatrists.

For over two decades, antiepileptic drugs (AEDs) have been integral to the treatment of bipolar illness. Historically, the introduction of AEDs into the pharmacopeia was a consequence of Robert Post and James Ballenger's translational work of the kindling hypothesis to the clinical setting (Ballenger and Post 1980). The initial studies with carbamazepine led to widespread use, particularly in Europe (Post et al. 1996) and paved the way to the subsequent introduction of valproic acid (Bowden et al. 1994). Several AEDs are now in widespread clinical use, with some being used as mood stabilizers while others are used for their anxiolytic (Pande et al. 1999, 2000b) or anorectic (Bray et al. 2003; Wilding et al. 2004) properties.

The expert consensus guidelines (Sachs et al. 2000) and the American Psychiatric Association bipolar treatment guideline (2002) both propose that lithium and mood-stabilizing AEDs be the first-line treatment for bipolar depression prior to the introduction of antidepressant medications. This chapter reviews the available research regarding the use of these agents in bipolar depression.

LITHIUM

Bipolar Depression

Lithium has been used for acute bipolar depression since its introduction for use in bipolar illness (El-Mallakh 1996). Controlled studies in bipolar patients invariably show significant improvement in the majority of acutely depressed bipolar patients (68%–100%, mean 68% response) (Goodwin et al. 1972; Mendels 1975). This is very similar to what might be expected of an antidepressant for unipolar illness (Stark and Hardison 1985), but is higher than the 51% efficacy rate of lithium in unipolar depression (El-Mallakh 1996). This clinically significant response rate stands in obvious contrast to general clinician experience with lithium. The discrepancy is explained by the fact that in the original controlled trials of lithium treatment, lithium levels were generally much higher (around 1.0 mM), than what is typically used by clinicians today (approximately 0.7 mM). There is ample evidence from lithium monotherapy studies (Gelenberg et al. 1989; Keller et al. 1992) and studies of lithium coadministration with an antidepressant (Nemeroff et al. 2001) that higher doses (and therefore blood levels) of lithium are more effective in treating and preventing depressive symptoms than lower doses. In their attempts to reduce the adverse-effect burden of lithium, clinicians are using it at doses that may be suboptimal for bipolar depression (El-Mallakh 1996).

Prophylaxis of Episodes

Lithium efficacy in preventing depressions in bipolar patients is not as clear. Early, long-term studies were not placebo-controlled, and have therefore been criticized regarding the methodology (Blackwell and Shepherd 1968). However, the best studies for the ability of lithium to prevent depressive relapse come from modern studies of lamotrigine, in which lithium is used as a positive control (Bowden et al. 2003; Calabrese et al. 2003; Goodwin et al. 2004). These studies are extraordinarily well designed, since minimum lithium serum levels were 0.8 mM or higher, and since they included patients that were either recently manic (Bowden et al. 2003) or recently depressed (Calabrese et al. 2003). This is an important characterization, since the polarity of the index episode appears to predict the polarity of the next episode (Calabrese et al. 2004), and thus the outcome is different for the two groups (Bowden et al. 2003; Calabrese et al. 2003). In these studies, a total of 638 patients were randomly assigned to treatment with lithium ($n=167$), lamotrigine ($n=280$), or placebo ($n=191$) and followed for 18 months. Outcome was need for intervention (not meeting DSM-IV criteria for an episode). Lithium was not effective in preventing depressive relapse in these patients compared with placebo (Goodwin et al. 2004).

LAMOTRIGINE

Bipolar Depression

Lamotrigine is an anticonvulsant with demonstrated efficacy in treating generalized and partial seizures (Bisulli et al. 2001; Brodie et al. 2002). It has been available for over 12 years but has only recently been investigated in bipolar illness. Nonetheless, because of its apparent efficacy in difficult-to-treat bipolar states (depression in both type I and type II patients and rapid cycling) its use has increased rapidly since its approval by the U.S. Food and Drug Administration (FDA). In a recent survey of participants in the large, National Institute of Mental Health (NIMH)–sponsored bipolar study (known as STEP-BD), 15% of bipolar patients were receiving lamotrigine (Marangell et al. 2004). Patients receiving lamotrigine were more likely to be rapid cycling or have had a history of an antidepressant-induced mania or hypomania (Marangell et al. 2004).

Two published trials have demonstrated the efficacy of lamotrigine monotherapy in depressed bipolar patients. The first of these, sponsored by the drug's manufacturer, was a double-blind, placebo-controlled, randomized, monotherapy trial of 195 depressed, type I, bipolar patients (Calabrese et al. 1999b). Two active arms administered lamotrigine at either 50 mg or 200 mg daily after a slow taper (50 mg was reached after 2 weeks, 200 mg was reached after 5 weeks). The study was designed with the primary outcome measure being improvement on the Hamilton Rating Scale for Depression (Ham-D). However, improvement did not reach statistical significance because of the high placebo response rate (37%) (Calabrese et al. 1999b). Nevertheless, participants' results on both the Clinical Global Impression (CGI) and the Montgomery-Åsberg Depression Rating Scale (MADRS) showed significant improvement at both 50-mg and 200-mg doses. For the MADRS the response rates were 54%, 48%, and 29% for lamotrigine 200 mg, lamotrigine 50 mg, and placebo, respectively. This effect size is similar to that seen for antidepressants in the treatment of unipolar depression (Stark and Hardison 1985). Despite the slow titration schedule, the lamotrigine groups separated from placebo at 3 weeks (1 week after reaching the 50-mg dose), and remained superior for the remaining 4 weeks of the study (Calabrese et al. 1999b).

Similar results were obtained in the second randomized, placebo-controlled trial when Frye et al. (2000) examined 31 severely ill, bipolar I subjects in a triple cross-over design (examining lamotrigine, gabapentin, and placebo). The response rate of 52% in the lamotrigine group was statistically superior to both gabapentin (26%), and placebo (23%) (Frye et al. 2000).

Prophylaxis of Episodes

Lamotrigine has been studied in two large, placebo-controlled, long-term (18-months), maintenance trials. These studies were designed to examine patients who had recently been manic (Bowden et al. 2003; Goodwin et al. 2004) and those who had recently been depressed (Calabrese et al. 2003; Goodwin et al. 2004). In both studies, lamotrigine was more effective at preventing or delaying future depressions than mania or hypomania. A combined analysis of 638 patients, who were randomized to one of three groups (lithium, lamotrigine, or placebo), found that both lithium and lamotrigine were superior to placebo at delaying intervention for depression and that lamotrigine was numerically superior to lithium (Goodwin et al. 2004). These studies have led to the approval of lamotrigine by the FDA for maintenance treatment in bipolar disorder.

Type II bipolar patients experienced a similar outcome in an open study in which lamotrigine was administered for 6 months to 17 patients (Vieta et al. 2003). Twelve patients completed the study (70%) and experienced a significant reduction in the Ham-D score and a significant improvement in the CGI score (Vieta et al. 2003).

Adjunctive Use

Lamotrigine may also be useful as an adjunct. In an open add-on, naturalistic study of 22 nonresponsive (to either divalproex plus and antidepressant or divalproex plus a mood stabilizer), depressed, bipolar subjects, lamotrigine was very effecitve (Kusumaker and Yatham 1997). Sixteen of the 22 subjects (72%) were responsive by the end of week 4. Suppes et al. (1999) reported a similar study with a similar outcome in which nine type I bipolar subjects and eight type II bipolar subjects who had not done well with other medications had lamotrigine added to their regimen. Eleven (65%) improved significantly over the 5-month observation period. Calabrese et al. (1999a) openly treated 15 patients with lamotrigine monotherapy and 60 patients with add-on lamotrigine for 48 weeks. Patients had type I or type II bipolar disorder, but only 40 were depressed when they entered the study. Forty-eight percent experienced marked improvement and an additional 20% had moderate improvement. In another study, lamotrigine or placebo were added to fluoxetine in eight type II bipolar patients who did not improve while receiving fluoxetine monotherapy (Barbosa et al. 2003). Although there was not a significant change in the Ham-D scores for this small study, the CGI scores improved in 84% of lamotrigine plus fluoxetine subjects, compared with 30% of fluoxetine-only subjects (Barbosa et al. 2003).

VALPROIC ACID

Bipolar Depression

Valproic acid (usually in the divalproex formulation) is the most widely used mood stabilizer in the treatment of bipolar disorder in the United States. This is due to the documented efficacy of the divalproex formulation in acute mania (Bowden et al. 1994) and effective marketing by Abbott Laboratories. Nevertheless, the utility of valproic acid in bipolar depression is not well characterized. The utility of divalproex in the depressive symptoms of acute mania (Swann et al. 1997) and mixed mania (Calabrese et al. 1992) has been generalized to include efficacy in bipolar depression.

Two blinded, controlled studies of valproic acid have been conducted using patients with bipolar depression. In one study, reported by Young et al. (2000), 11 type I and 16 type II bipolar disorder patients were randomly assigned to receive paroxetine or a mood stabilizer in addition to lithium or divalproex. Sixteen patients were randomized to receive two mood stabilizers and 11 received a combination of lithium or divalproex plus paroxetine. Combined mood stabilizer therapy was generally poorly tolerated, and six of the patients did not complete the 6-week trial. For the remaining patients, there were no differences in the outcomes between the two groups and everybody improved (Young et al. 2000). However, in a small ($n=43$), unpublished, blinded, placebo-controlled, 2-month study of divalproex in acutely depressed bipolar subjects, there was no significant difference between placebo and divalproex (20.5- vs. 22.6-point improvement on the Ham-D) (G. Sachs, per-

At least one study shows that divalproex may be more effective in depressed type II bipolar patients. In an open, 12-week, monotherapy study of medication-naïve ($n=11$) or mood stabilizer–naïve ($n=8$, treated previously with antidepressants or stimulants) bipolar II patients, 63% of patients were considered responders (>50% decrease on Ham-D scores) (Winsberg et al. 2001). This result was due primarily to medication-naïve patients doing very well (82% response rate), whereas mood stabilizer–naïve patients did poorly (38% response rate).

Adjunctive Use

Combining divalproex with lithium appears to be as effective as adding an antidepressant to either lithium or divalproex in acutely depressed bipolar patients (Young et al. 2000). In a 6-week, double-blind, add-on comparison examining two mood stabilizers with a single mood stabilizer and an antidepressant in acutely depressed type I ($n=11$) and type II ($n=16$) bipolar subjects, all subjects improved to an equal degree (Young et al. 2000). However, the combination mood stabilizer group had a high rate of dropouts (37.5%; two secondary to inadequate response, two due to poor compliance, one due to emergence of a mixed state, and one due to unrelated medical problem) compared with the antidepressant plus mood stabilizer group (0%) suggesting that combination mood stabilizers are relatively poorly tolerated.

The combination of valproic acid with an antipsychotic appears to be more effective than divalproex alone. Tohen et al. (2002) reported the addition of olanzapine or placebo to lithium or valproic acid in the treatment of 344 patients with type I bipolar disorder who were experiencing a manic or mixed manic episode. In a subanalysis of 85 patients who had a Ham-D score of 20 or more, the improvement in depressive symptoms was significantly greater in those treated with a combination than those treated with monotherapy (Baker et al. 2004). However, as noted above, efficacy in dysphoria associated with mania does not mean efficacy in bipolar depression.

Prophylaxis of Episodes

Long-term use of divalproex in maintenance treatment of bipolar illness has been studied in both open and controlled fashions. Bowden et al. (2000) reported a 1-year study of recently manic bipolar subjects (defined by DSM-III-R) assigned to divalproex, lithium, or placebo. There were no differences from any of the three groups regarding the primary outcome measure of time to any mood episode. Importantly, there was no difference between lithium and placebo in this study. Since lithium is essentially a positive control, its lack of efficacy in this study indicates that the study failed and that the data are not reliable. The reasons this study failed are not clear; but they may be related to the utilization of DSM-III-R criteria, which are different from the Research Diagnostic Criteria utilized in the initial divalproex study (Bowden et al. 1994), and subsequent DSM-IV studies. Nonetheless, secondary analyses have been performed on these data. In addition to the fact that the long-term divalproex study failed, there is an additional problem with its data regarding bipolar depression. Utilizing a sample of recently manic patients is suboptimal for investigating relapse into depression because the polarity of the most recent episode predicts polarity of the subsequent episode (Calabrese et al. 2004)—meaning that these study participants were less likely to relapse into mania. However, Bowden et al. (2005) examined the outcome as a function of the type of mania of the index episode (i.e., euphoric [$n=123$] versus dysphoric [$n=249$]) and in this subanalysis, divalproex was significantly superior to lithium (but not placebo) in delaying time to depressive relapse. Furthermore, divalproex was superior to lithium in longer duration of successful prophylaxis and better depressive symptom scores (Bowden et al. 2000; Gyulai et al. 2003). Among patients who were placed on an antidepressant during the study, those on concomitant divalproex treatment were less likely to drop out of the study (Gyulai et al. 2003). Prior response to divalproex appeared to predict a subsequently lower rate of relapse into depression (Gyulai et al. 2003).

Eli Lilly and Company sponsored a 47-week, blinded, comparison, relapse-prevention trial in 251 type I patients (Tohen et al. 2003). The patients entered the study with acute mania or mixed mania and were treated with divalproex (500–2,500 mg/day) or olanzapine (5–20 mg/day). Over the 47 weeks, olanzapine and divalproex were equally effective (although olanzapine improved the mania faster) and there were no differences in the relapse rates into mania or depression, although the relapse rates were high for both agents used in monotherapy (56.8% for olanzapine and 45.5% for divalproex) (Tohen et al. 2003). When an accepted mood stabilizer (lithium or divalproex) was combined with olanzapine, relapse into depression was nonsignificantly delayed compared with a mood stabilizer alone in a randomized, blinded study (55 vs. 163 days, $P=0.07$) (Tohen et al. 2004).

Several naturalistic studies suggest that divalproex is useful in relapse prevention. In an open, 15-month, prospective study of 78 patients with rapid-cycling bipolar disorder, 30 patients were treated with monotherapy and 48 patients received divalproex added to other psychotropics (Calabrese et al. 1992; this study was an extension of a previous publication, Calabrese and Delucchi 1990). Response rates for mixed manic episodes were quite high at 87%, mania improved in 54%, but only 19% of those with depression were responsive. Hayes (1989) reported on 12 bipolar subjects who started divalproex as an add-on medication when significantly symptomatic. After 1 year they experienced an average of 27.7 points improvement on the Global Assessment of Functioning (GAF) (Hayes 1989).

An interesting study was performed in a group of 30 women who had type II bipolar illness and borderline personality disorder (Frankenburg and Zanarini 2002). The patients were assigned to divalproex or placebo in a 2:1 ratio. Patients receiving divalproex experienced significantly greater improvement in irritability, anger, impulsive aggression, and interpersonal sensitivity (Frankenburg and Zanarini 2002). This is similar to what was observed in an open, 8-week study of 11 patients with borderline personality disorder (without bipolar illness). Only eight patients completed the study and, of these, only three responded with a reduction in anger, impulsivity, rejection sensitivity, and anxiety. Fifty percent of completers experienced an improvement in mood (Stein et al. 1995).

Combining divalproex with lithium for relapse prevention has also been examined in open studies. Random assignment to lithium alone or lithium plus divalproex was studied (using DSM-III-R criteria) in 20 bipolar patients who were followed for 1 year in an open fashion: receiving combination treatments resulted in a significantly lower risk for relapse but a higher incidence of adverse events (Solomon et al. 1997). Similarly, when a group of rapid-cycling bipolar patients treated with lithium plus divalproex were followed for 6 months, 60% experienced marked antidepressant efficacy, and 50% experienced bimodal (antidepressant and antimanic) efficacy (Calabrese et al. 2001). Nonetheless, when these patients relapsed, the relapse was usually depressive (Calabrese et al. 2001).

In summary, valproic acid appears to be quite effective in reducing the depressive symptoms associated with acute mixed mania, but less than desirable in its antidepressive effect in depressed bipolar patients. It also appears to be suboptimal in its ability to prevent relapse into bipolar depression, although it is not without efficacy. The data for valproic acid are educational in that it is clear that efficacy in the depressive symptoms of mania does not predict efficacy in bipolar depression. The two states appear to be biologically different and respond to different treatments.

CARBAMAZEPINE

Bipolar Depression

Carbamazepine is the first anticonvulsant to demonstrate efficacy in the treatment of bipolar illness but only recently received FDA approval after Shire Pharmaceuticals pursued large, placebo-controlled studies of its use in acute mania (Weisler et al. 2004, 2005). Interestingly, it has demonstrated moderate efficacy in animal models of depression (Barros and Leite 1987) as well as human unipolar depression in both double-blind studies (Post et al. 1986) and small open trials (Dietrich and Emrich 1998; Kudoh et al. 1998; Steinacher et al. 2002).

The first placebo-controlled study to be performed with carbamazepine in bipolar illness included treatment of 13 depressed bipolar subjects (Ballenger and Post 1980). Five (38.5%) experienced significant improvement, and three relapsed when switched to placebo. Although several other controlled studies have been performed with carbamazepine, they often included both bipolar and unipolar depressed individuals (usually treatment-resistant patients). However, when the four controlled studies and eight open studies are combined, the overall response rate of depression to carbamazepine is 55% (Post et al. 1996).

The largest study was a 3-week open administration of carbamazepine to 27 depressed bipolar outpatients. The Ham-D score declined by a mean of 23.7 points over the 3 weeks and 17 patients (63%) entered into remission (Dilsaver et al. 1996). Although open studies generally overestimate true response rates, the extraordinarily positive outcome of this study suggests a true antidepressant action of carbamazepine in bipolar depression.

In a survey of 9,030 physician members of the American Psychiatric Association, among the 28% (2,543) who responded, carbamazepine was judged to be effective in 67.5% of bipolar depressed patients but only 32.2% of unipolar depressed patients (Denicoff et al. 1994). Only about 4.4% of patients needed to be withdrawn from carbamazepine because of adverse effects (Denicoff et al. 1994).

Although the mechanism of action in carbamazepine for bipolar depression is unknown, the only biological measure that has been found to be significantly related to the degree of symptomatic improvement is the concentration of the 10,11-epoxide metabolite in the cerebrospinal fluid (Post et al. 1983). This would suggest that the antidepressant effect of carbamazepine is unique to this agent and cannot be generalized to the related compound, oxcarbazepine, which does not have a 10,11-epoxide metabolite.

Prophylaxis of Episodes

The prophylactic efficacy of carbamazepine was examined in two prospective, randomized trials. In a 3-year, random-assignment study of 83 DSM-III–defined bipolar patients placed on lithium or carbamazepine, efficacy of the agents was found to be equivalent and better at prevention of manias and hypomanias (Placidi et al. 1986). In another study, in which 52 DSM-III–defined bipolar subjects were randomly crossed over to lithium or carbamazepine monotherapy or the two agents combined, the two monotherapies were found to be equivalent in efficacy, but combination treatment was nearly twice as effective (Denicoff et al. 1997).

A 2.5-year, naturalist, follow-up study of 114 patients treated with either lithium or carbamazepine alone found that lithium was superior to carbamazepine overall. However, subjects with nonclassic bipolar illness (e.g., with type II disorder or with mixed manias or rapid-cycling course) tended to do better with carbamazepine (Kleindienst and Greil 2000). A similar response was noted in an open, long-term follow-up of 32 bipolar subjects treated with carbamazepine: those with atypical symptoms (e.g., earlier age at onset or continuous symptoms rather than episodic) showed having experienced the greatest benefit (Kishimoto et al. 1983).

Some studies have shown that there may be a fade effect with carbamazepine. In a 2-year study of 24 treatment-resistant bipolar subjects, response rates decreased from 72% in the first year to 66% in the second year (Post et al. 1990). About half of the patients ($n=11$) experienced loss of prophylaxis in the second year (Post et al. 1990). When carbamazepine was combined with divalproex, bipolar subjects (but not schizoaffective patients) appeared to do well in a retrospective analysis (Tohen et al. 1994).

OXCARBAZEPINE

Despite being poorly studied with respect to bipolar illness, oxcarbazepine has made it into the American Psychiatric Association practice guideline for bipolar treatment (2002). Its utility in bipolar depression is even more poorly studied than in mania and hypomania. The observation that oxcarbazepine reverses abnormal behavior in two rat models of depression (Beijamini et al. 1998) suggests that it may indeed have antidepressant properties. In a group of 56 bipolar patients presenting with depression ($n=23$), mania ($n=19$), or psychosis ($n=14$), there were no differences in outcome between any of the groups, suggesting that the study measures were inadequate. Twenty percent experienced no clear benefit (Centorrino et al. 2003). As noted earlier, the antidepressant effect of carbamazepine has been associated with the cerebrospinal fluid concentrations of the 10,11-epoxide metabolite (Post et al. 1983). Since oxcarbazepine does not have that metabolite, it may also lack an antidepressant effect in bipolar illness.

TOPIRAMATE

Topiramate is an anticonvulsant with several interesting properties (Yen et al. 2000): it is associated with weight loss, may be an effective anti-obesity agent (Bray et al. 2003; Wilding et al. 2004), and may actually increase insulin sensitivity (Wilkes et al. 2005a, 2005b), possibly making it useful in the management of weight gain and obesity, which frequently accompany bipolar disorder (McElroy et al. 2004). Furthermore, topiramate may be effective in reducing binge-eating behavior (McElroy et al. 2003), bulimia (Hedges et al. 2003; Hoopes et al. 2003), and alcohol consumption (Johnson et al. 2003). For these reasons, topiramate is a frequently used drug in bipolar patients. However, initial reports that topiramate is an effective mood stabilizer have not been borne out by more extensive double-blind, placebo-controlled studies. Unfortunately, many of these reports remain unpublished and therefore cannot be critically reviewed.

Two studies have been performed with topiramate in depressed bipolar subjects. In one, 36 patients with either type I or II bipolar disorder were randomly assigned to receive either topiramate or bupropion slow release added to current medication. Fifty-six percent of topiramate-treated patients and 59% of bupropion-treated patients improved at least 50% on the Ham-D (McIntyre et al. 2002). In an unpublished study, Hussain et al. (2001) studied long-term (3-year) topiramate use in 65 depressed type I and 18 depressed type II bipolar subjects. Sixty-three percent of the patients achieved remission (Ham-D<10) by the end of the study.

OTHER ANTICONVULSANTS

Few of the other available anticonvulsants have been studied in bipolar depression. Not all anticonvulsants have mood-stabilizing properties and fewer have an antidepressant effect.

Gabapentin

Gabapentin is an anticonvulsant with clinically meaningful efficacy in blinded, placebo-controlled studies in panic disorder (Pande et al. 2000b) and generalized anxiety disorder (Pande et al. 1999). Because of its anxiolytic effect and initial open series suggesting utility as a mood stabilizer (Altshuler et al. 1999; Cabras et al. 1999; Perugi et al. 1999, 2002), it has been widely used in bipolar patients. However, its poor performance in blinded, placebo-controlled monotherapy (Frye et al. 2000) and adjunct studies (in which it was statistically inferior to placebo; Pande et al. 2000a) suggests that it has a limited role in acute mania. Nonetheless, with efficacy in different types of anxiety disorders, the question remains of whether gabapentin can be effective in bipolar depression.

In the only placebo-controlled study that utilized a crossover design, 31 treatment-resistant bipolar patients did not experience any benefit from gabapentin compared with placebo in the treatment of depressive symptoms (Frye et al. 2000; Obrocea et al. 2002). However, positive responses have been reported in open trials. For example, Vieta and collegues (2000) found that 8 of 22 type I and II bipolar subjects with residual symptoms (36.4%) had a good response, particularly in anxious symptoms. Wang et al. (2002) found that 50% of 22 depressed type I ($n=10$) and type II ($n=12$) bipolar subjects experienced a moderate to marked improvement when gabapentin was added to a mood stabilizer or an antipsychotic agent. Eight (36%) achieved remission: the more mildly depressed subjects were the ones that improved and severely ill subjects did not do well (Wang et al. 2002). Perugi et al. (2002) gave gabapentin to 43 treatment-resistant DSM-III bipolar subjects. Eighteen (42%) responded and 17 of these subjects maintained the response for a full year. But the greatest improvement was experienced by those with anxiety, somatization, and alcohol abuse (Perugi et al. 2002). Ghaemi and Goodwin (2001) reviewed the records of 21 bipolar spectrum subjects treated with gabapentin (13 receiving monotherapy). They found that overall improvement in depressive symptoms was 27.6%. A subgroup with greater response (57.5% improvement) did not achieve statistical significance ($P=0.1$). Overall, these open studies are associated with placebo-like rates of response (30%–40% range) and improvement in mild or anxious symptoms, suggesting that gabapentin is not generally helpful in bipolar depression but may be helpful in mildly depressed, anxious individuals. A similar conclusion was reached in a more extensive review of the open data (Carta et al. 2003).

A similar pattern is seen when patients have mild mixed symptoms.

Sokolski et al. (1999) and Young et al. (1999) both reported a significant decrease in symptoms of hypomania and depression in mildly ill type I or type II bipolar disorder patients. Again, anxiety symptoms were not specifically measured, but may have accounted for most of the improvement.

More clear is the lack of prophylactic effect of gabapentin in long-term treatment. Montanes Rada and de Lucas Taracena (2001) openly followed nine bipolar patients receiving gabapentin monotherapy for 9 months. Overall the patients did worse after beginning gabapentin, with an increase in the number of relapses (from an average of 0.18/month to 0.29/month). Similarly, in another study of 18 patients with an initial good response to gabapentin, only seven (39%) experienced ongoing benefit, while five relapsed (three dropped out) (Schaffer and Schaffer 1999).

Tiagabine

Tiagabine is an approved antiepileptic agent (Sachdeo et al. 1997). Suppes and colleagues in the Stanley Bipolar Network (2002) examined tiagabine at an average dose of 8.7 mg/day in 17 refractory bipolar patients. Only three (23%) improved, the majority (77%) either experienced no change or worsened. Similarly, Schaffer et al. (2002) reported a small open series of 22 bipolar spectrum patients who received low-dose tiagabine (<8 mg/day) as an add-on to other mood stabilizers. At the end of 6 months only eight (36%) were considered responders.

Pregabalin

Pregabalin is an antiepileptic compound related to gabapentin (Arroyo et al. 2004) that has significant anxiolytic effect in generalized anxiety disorder (Feltner et al. 2003; Pande et al. 2003; Pary 2004) and social phobia (Pande et al. 2004). Bipolar studies are unpublished and are believed to be negative.

Levetiracetam

Levetiracetam is an antiepileptic agent (Cereghino et al. 2000) that has been preliminarily examined in depressed bipolar subjects. Post et al. (2005) described that only 31% of depressed patients had significant improvement after 8 weeks of treatment with 2,000–3,000 mg/day. The low response rates suggest that additional preliminary studies are still required.

SUMMARY

Lithium and anticonvulsants have a significant role in the treatment of bipolar depression. Lithium has extensive data supporting its utility in both acute bipolar depression and relapse prevention. Additionally, it has well-documented anti-suicide potency. Lamotrigine has been shown in placebo-controlled trials to improve acute depression and prevent depressive relapse in both types I and II bipolar subjects. Valproic acid has not been adequately studied in acute bipolar depression, and available evidence indicates suboptimal benefit. However, secondary analyses of a controlled relapse prevention study and open data suggest that it may have a role in the delay or prevention of depressive episodes in bipolar patients. Carbamazepine appears to have a modest acute and prophylactic antidepressant effect. Other agents have not been adequately studied in bipolar depression but may improve other associated symptoms (e.g., anxiety with gabapentin) to play a role in the management of bipolar depression.

REFERENCES

Altshuler LL, Keck PE Jr, McElroy SL, et al: Gabapentin in the acute treatment of refractory bipolar disorder. Bipolar Disord 1:61–65, 1999

American Psychiatric Association: Practice guideline for the treatment of patients with bipolar disorder (revision). Work Group on Bipolar Disorder. Am J Psychiatry 159(suppl):1–50, 2002

Arroyo S, Anhut H, Kugler AR, et al: Pregabalin add-on treatment: a randomized, double-blind, placebo-controlled, dose-response study in adults with partial seizures. Epilepsia 45:20–27, 2004

Baker RW, Brown E, Akiskal HS, et al: Efficacy of olanzapine combined with valproate or lithium in treatment of dysphoric mania. Br J Psychiatry 185:472–478, 2004

Ballenger JC, Post RM: Carbamazepine in manic-depressive illness: a new treatment. Am J Psychiatry 137:782–790, 1980

Barbosa L, Berk M, Vorster M: A double-blind, randomized, placebo-controlled trial of augmentation with lamotrigine or placebo in patients concomitantly treated with fluoxetine for resistant major depressive episodes. J Clin Psychiatry 64:403–407, 2003

Barros HM, Leite JR: The effects of carbamazepine on two animal models of depression. Psychopharmacology (Berl) 92:340–342, 1987

Beijamini V, Skalisz LL, Joca SR, et al: The effect of oxcarbazepine on behavioural despair and learned helplessness. Eur J Pharmacol 347:23–27, 1998

Bisulli F, Baruzzi A, Rosati A, et al: Efficacy of lamotrigine add-on therapy in severe partial epilepsy in adults with drop seizures and secondary bilateral synchrony on EEG. Epileptic Disord 3:151–156, 2001

Blackwell B, Shepherd M: Prophylactic lithium: another therapeutic myth? An examination of the evidence to date. Lancet 1:968–971, 1968

Bowden CL, Brugger AM, Swann AC, et al: Efficacy of divalproex vs. lithium and placebo in the treatment of mania. The Depakote Mania Study Group. J Am Med Assoc 271:918–924, 1994

Bowden CL, Calabrese JR, McElroy SL, et al: A randomized, placebo-controlled 12-month trial of divalproex and lithium in the treatment of outpatients with bipolar I disorder. Divalproex Maintenance Study Group. Arch Gen Psychiatry 57:481–489, 2000

Bowden CL, Calabrese JR, Sachs G, et al: A placebo-controlled 18-month trial of lamotrigine and lithium maintenance treatment in recently manic or hypomanic patients with bipolar I disorder. Arch Gen Psychiatry 60:392–400, 2003

Bowden CL, Collins MA, McElroy SL, et al: Relationship of mania symptomatology to maintenance treatment response with divalproex, lithium, or placebo. Neuropsychopharmacol 30:1932–1939, 2005

Bray GA, Hollander P, Klein S, et al: A 6-month randomized, placebo-controlled, dose-ranging trial of topiramate for weight loss in obesity. Obes Res 11:722–733, 2003

Brodie MJ, Chadwick DW, Anhut H, et al: Gabapentin versus lamotrigine monotherapy: a double-blind comparison in newly diagnosed epilepsy. Epilepsia 43:993–1000, 2002

Cabras PL, Hardoy MJ, Hardoy MC, et al: Clinical experience with gabapentin in patients with bipolar or schizoaffective disorder: results of an open-label study. J Clin Psychiatry 60:245–248, 1999

Calabrese JR, Delucchi GA: Spectrum of efficacy of valproate in 55 patients with rapid-cycling bipolar disorder. Am J Psychiatry 147:431–434, 1990

Calabrese JR, Markovitz PJ, Kimmel SE, et al: Spectrum of efficacy of valproate in 78 rapid-cycling bipolar patients. J Clin Psychopharmacol 12 (suppl 1):53S–56S, 1992

Calabrese JR, Bowden CL, McElroy SL, et al: Spectrum of activity of lamotrigine in treatment-refractory bipolar disorder. Am J Psychiatry 156:1019–1023, 1999a

Calabrese JR, Bowden CL, Sachs GS, et al: A double-blind placebo-controlled study of lamotrigine monotherapy in outpatients with bipolar I depression. Lamictal 602 Study Group. J Clin Psychiatry 60:79–88, 1999b

Calabrese JR, Shelton MD, Bowden CL, et al: Bipolar rapid cycling: focus on depression as its hallmark. J Clin Psychiatry 62 (suppl 14):34–41, 2001

Calabrese JR, Bowden CL, Sachs GS, et al: A placebo-controlled 18-month trial of lamotrigine and lithium maintenance treatment in recently depressed patients with bipolar I disorder. J Clin Psychiatry 64:1013–1024, 2003

Calabrese JR, Vieta E, El-Mallakh, RS, et al: Mood state at study entry as predictor of relapse risk and efficacy spectrum. Biol Psychiatry 56:957–963, 2004

Carta MG, Hardoy MC, Hardoy MJ, et al: The clinical use of gabapentin in bipolar spectrum disorders. J Affect Disord 75:83–91, 2003

Centorrino F, Albert MJ, Berry JM, et al: Oxcarbazepine: clinical experience with hospitalized psychiatric patients. Bipolar Disord 5:370–374, 2003

Cereghino JJ, Biton V, Abou-Khalil B, et al: Levetiracetam for partial seizures: results of a double-blind, randomized clinical trial. Neurology 55:236–242, 2000

Denicoff KD, Meglathery SB, Post RM, et al: Efficacy of carbamazepine compared with other agents: a clinical practice survey. J Clin Psychiatry 55:70–76, 1994

Denicoff KD, Smith-Jackson EE, Disney ER, et al: Comparative prophylactic efficacy of lithium, carbamazepine, and the combination in bipolar disorder. J Clin Psychiatry 58:470–478, 1997

Dietrich DE, Emrich HM: The use of anticonvulsants to augment antidepressant medication. J Clin Psychiatry 59 (suppl 5):51–58, 1998

Dilsaver SC, Swann SC, Chen YW, et al: Treatment of bipolar depression with carbamazepine: results of an open study. Biol Psychiatry 40:935–937, 1996

El-Mallakh RS: Lithium: Actions and Mechanisms. Washington, DC, American Psychiatric Press, 1996

Feltner DE, Crockatt JG, Dubovsky SJ, et al: A randomized, double-blind, placebo-controlled, fixed-dose, multicenter study of pregabalin in patients with generalized anxiety disorder. J Clin Psychopharmacol 23:240–249, 2003

Frankenburg FR, Zanarini MC: Divalproex sodium treatment of women with borderline personality disorder and bipolar II disorder: a double-blind, placebo-controlled pilot study. J Clin Psychiatry 63:442–446, 2002

Frye MA, Ketter TA, Kimbrell TA, et al: A placebo-controlled study of lamotrigine and gabapentin monotherapy in refractory mood disorders. J Clin Psychopharmacol 20:607–614, 2000

Gelenberg AJ, Kane JM, Keller MB, et al: Comparison of standard and low serum levels of lithium for maintenance treatment of bipolar disorder. N Engl J Med 321:1489–1493, 1989

Ghaemi SN, Goodwin FK: Gabapentin treatment of the non-refractory bipolar spectrum: an open case series. J Affect Disord 65:167–171, 2001

Goodwin FK, Murphy DL, Dunner DL, et al: Lithium response in unipolar vs. bipolar depression. Am J Psychiatry 129:44–47, 1972

Goodwin GM, Bowden CL, Calabrese JR, et al: A pooled analysis of 2 placebo-controlled 18-month trials of lamotrigine and lithium maintenance in bipolar I disorder. J Clin Psychiatry 65:432–441, 2004

Gyulai L, Bowden CL, McElroy SL, et al: Maintenance efficacy of divalproex in the prevention of bipolar depression. Neuropsychopharmacol 28:1374–1382, 2003

Hayes SG: Long-term use of valproate in primary psychiatric disorders. J Clin Psychiatry 50(suppl):35–39, 1989

Hedges DW, Reimherr FW, Hoopes SP, et al: Treatment of bulimia nervosa with topiramate in a randomized, double-blind, placebo-controlled trial, part 2: improvement in psychiatric measures. J Clin Psychiatry 64:1449–1454, 2003

Hoopes SP, Reimherr FW, Hedges DW, et al: Treatment of bulimia nervosa with topiramate in a randomized, double-blind, placebo-controlled trial, part 1: improvement in binge and purge measures. J Clin Psychiatry 64:1335–1341, 2003

Hussain MZ, Chaudhry ZA, Hussain S: Topiramate in treatment of refractory bipolar depression (poster abstract). Bipolar Disord 3:43, 2001

Johnson BA, Ait-Daoud N, Bowden CL, et al: Oral topiramate in the treatment of alcohol dependence: a randomised controlled trial. Lancet 361: 1677–1685, 2003

Keller MB, Lavori PW, Kane JM, et al: Subsyndromal symptoms in bipolar disorder: a comparison of standard and low serum levels of lithium. Arch Gen Psychiatry 49:371–376, 1992

Kishimoto A, Ogura C, Hazama H, et al: Long-term prophylactic effects of carbamazepine in affective disorder. Br J Psychiatry 143:327–331, 1983

Kleindienst N, Greil W: Differential efficacy of lithium and carbamazepine in the prophylaxis of bipolar disorder: results of the MAP study. Neuropsychobiology 42(suppl):2–10, 2000

Kudoh A, Ishihara H, Matsuki A: Effect of carbamazepine on pain scores of unipolar depressed patients with chronic pain: a trial of off-on-off design. Clin J Pain 14:61–65, 1998

Kusumaker V, Yatham LN: An open study of lamotrigine in refractory bipolar depression. Psychiatry Res 72:145–148, 1997

Marangell LB, Martinez JM, Ketter TA, et al: Lamotrigine treatment of bipolar disorder: data from the first 500 patients in STEP-BD. Bipolar Disord 6:139–143, 2004

McElroy SL, Arnold LM, Shapira NA, et al: Topiramate in the treatment of binge eating disorder associated with obesity: a randomized, placebo-controlled trial. Am J Psychiatry 160:255–261, 2003; erratum 160:612, 2003

McElroy SL, Kotwal R, Malhotra S, et al: Are mood disorders and obesity related? A review for the mental health professional. J Clin Psychiatry 65:634–651, 2004

McIntyre RS, Mancini DA, McCann S, et al: Topiramate versus bupropion SR when added to mood stabilizer therapy for the depressive phase of bipolar disorder: a preliminary single blind study. Bipolar Disord 4:207–213, 2002

Mendels J: Lithium in the acute treatment of depressive states, in Lithium Research and Therapy. Edited by Johnson FN. London, Academic Press, 1975, pp 43–62

Montanes Rada F, de Lucas Taracena MT: Efficacy of gabapentin in a sample of bipolar patients [in Spanish]. Acta Esp Psiquiatr 29:386–389, 2001

Nemeroff CB, Evans DL, Gyulai L, et al: A double-blind, placebo-controlled comparison of imipramine and paroxetine in the treatment of bipolar depression. Am J Psychiatry 158:906–912, 2001

Obrocea GV, Dunn RM, Frye MA, et al: Clinical predictors of response to lamotrigine and gabapentin monotherapy in refractory affective disorders. Biol Psychiatry 51:253–260, 2002

Pande AC, Davidson JR, Jefferson JW, et al: Treatment of social phobia with gabapentin: a placebo-controlled study. J Clin Psychopharmacol 19:341–348, 1999

Pande AC, Crockatt JG, Janney CA, et al: Gabapentin in bipolar disorder: a placebo-controlled trial of adjunctive therapy. Gabapentin Bipolar Disorder Study Group. Bipolar Disord 2:249–255, 2000a

Pande AC, Pollack MH, Crockatt J, et al: Placebo-controlled study of gabapentin treatment of panic disorder. J Clin Psychopharmacol 20:467–471, 2000b

Pande AC, Crockatt JG, Feltner DE, et al: Pregabalin in generalized anxiety disorder: a placebo-controlled trial. Am J Psychiatry 160:533–540, 2003

Pande AC, Feltner DE, Jefferson JW, et al: Efficacy of the novel anxiolytic pregabalin in social anxiety disorder: a placebo-controlled, multicenter study. J Clin Psychopharmacol 24:141–149, 2004

Pary R: High dose pregabalin is effective for the treatment of generalised anxiety disorder. Evid Based Ment Health 7:17, 2004

Perugi G, Toni C, Ruffalo G, et al: Clinical experience using adjunctive gabapentin in treatment-resistant bipolar mixed states. Pharmacopsychiatry 32:136–141, 1999

Perugi G, Toni C, Frare F, et al: Effectiveness of adjunctive gabapentin in resistant bipolar disorder: is it due to anxious-alcohol abuse comorbidity? Clin Psychopharmacol 22:584–591, 2002

Placidi GF, Lenzi A, Lazzerini F, et al: The comparative efficacy and safety of carbamazepine versus lithium: a randomized, double-blind 3-year trial in 83 patients. J Clin Psychiatry 47:490–494, 1986

Post RM, Uhde TW, Ballenger JC, et al: Carbamazepine and its -10,11-epoxide metabolite in plasma and CSF. Relationship to antidepressant response. Arch Gen Psychiatry 40:673–676, 1983

Post RM, Uhde TW, Roy-Byrne PP, et al: Antidepressant effects of carbamazepine. Am J Psychiatry 143:29–34, 1986

Post RM, Leverich GS, Rosoff AS, et al: Carbamazepine prophylaxis in refractory affective disorders: focus on long-term follow-up. J Clin Psychopharmacol 10:318–327, 1990

Post RM, Ketter TA, Denicoff K, et al: The place of anticonvulsant therapy in bipolar illness. Psychopharmacol (Berl) 128:115–129, 1996

Post RM, Altshuler LL, Frye MA, et al: Preliminary observations on the effectiveness of levetiracetam in the open adjunctive treatment of refractory bipolar disorder. J Clin Psychiatry 66:370–374, 2005

Sachdeo RC, Leroy RF, Krauss GL, et al: Tiagabine therapy for complex partial seizures. A dose-frequency study. The Tiagabine Study Group. Arch Neurol 54:595–601, 1997

Sachs GS, Printz DJ, Kahn DA, et al: The expert consensus guidelines series: medication treatment of bipolar disorder 2000. Postgrad Med Spec No:1–104, 2000

Schaffer CB, Schaffer LC: Open maintenance treatment of bipolar disorder spectrum patients who responded to gabapentin augmentation in the acute phase of treatment. J Affect Disord 55:237–240, 1999

Schaffer LC, Schaffer CB, Howe J: An open case series on the utility of tiagabine as an augmentation in refractory bipolar outpatients. J Affect Disord 71:259–263, 2002

Schou M: Lithium treatment at 52. J Affect Disord 67:21–32, 2001

Sokolski KN, Green C, Maris DE, et al: Gabapentin as an adjunct to standard mood stabilizers in outpatients with mixed bipolar symptomatology. Ann Clin Psychiatry 11:217–222, 1999

Solomon DA, Ryan CE, Keitner GI, et al: A pilot study of lithium carbonate plus divalproex sodium for continuation and maintenance treatment of patients with bipolar disorder. J Clin Psychiatry 58:95–99, 1997

Stark P, Hardison CD: A review of multicenter controlled studies of fluoxetine vs. imipramine and placebo in outpatients with major depressive disorder. J Clin Psychiatry 46:53–58, 1985

Stein DJ, Simeon D, Frenkel M, et al: An open trial of valproate in borderline personality disorder. J Clin Psychiatry 56:506–510, 1995

Steinacher L, Vandel P, Zullino DF, et al: Carbamazepine augmentation in depressive patients non-responding to citalopram: a pharmacokinetic and clinical pilot study. Eur Neuropsychopharmacol 12:255–260, 2002

Suppes T, Brown ES, McElroy SL, et al: Lamotrigine for the treatment of bipolar disorder: a clinical case series. J Affect Disord 53:95–98, 1999

Suppes T, Chisholm KA, Dhavale D, et al: Tiagabine in treatment refractory bipolar disorder: a clinical series. Bipolar Disord 4:283–289, 2002

Swann AC, Bowden CC, Morris D, et al: Depression during mania. Treatment response to lithium or divalproex. Arch Gen Psychiatry 54:37–42, 1997

Tohen M, Castillo J, Pope HG Jr, et al: Concomitant use of valproate and carbamazepine in bipolar and schizoaffective disorders. J Clin Psychopharmacol 14:67–70, 1994

Tohen M, Chengappa K, Suppes T, et al: Efficacy of olanzapine in combination with valproate or lithium in the treatment of mania in patients partially nonresponsive to valproate or lithium monotherapy. Arch Gen Psychiatry 59:62–69, 2002

Tohen M, Ketter TA, Zarate CA, et al: Olanzapine versus divalproex sodium for the treatment of acute mania and maintenance of remission: a 47-week study. Am J Psychiatry 160:1263–1271, 2003

Tohen M, Chengappa KN, Suppes T, et al: Relapse prevention in bipolar I disorder: 18-month comparison of olanzapine plus mood stabiliser v. mood stabiliser alone. Br J Psychiatry 184:337–345, 2004

Vieta E, Martinez-Aran A, Nieto E, et al: Adjunctive gabapentin treatment of bipolar disorder. Eur Psychiatry 15:433–437, 2000

Vieta E, Goikolea M, Benabarre A, et al: Treatment of bipolar II disorder with lamotrigine [in Spanish]. Acta Exp Psiquiatr 31:65–68, 2003

Wang PW, Santosa C, Schumacher M, et al: Gabapentin augmentation therapy in bipolar depression. Bipolar Disord 4:296–301, 2002

Weisler RH, Kalali AH, Ketter TA, et al: A multicenter, randomized, double-blind, placebo-controlled trial of extended-release carbamazepine capsules as monotherapy for bipolar disorder patients with manic or mixed episodes. J Clin Psychiatry 65:478–484, 2004

Weisler RH, Keck PE, Jr, Swann AC, et al: Extended-release carbamazepine capsules as monotherapy for acute mania in bipolar disorder: a multi-center, randomized, double-blind, placebo-controlled trial. J Clin Psychiatry 66:323–330, 2005

Wilding J, Van Gaal L, Rissanen A, et al: A randomized double-blind placebo-controlled study of the long term efficacy and safety of topiramate in the treatment of obese subjects. Int J Obes Relat Metab Disord 28:1399–1410, 2004

Wilkes JJ, Nelson E, Osborne M, et al: Topiramate is an insulin-sensitizing compound in vivo with direct effects on adipocytes in female ZDF rats. Am J Physiol Endocrinol Metab 288:E617–E624, 2005a

Wilkes JJ, Nguyen MT, Bandyopadhyay GK, et al: Topiramate treatment causes skeletal muscle insulin sensitization and increased Acrp30 secretion in high-fat-fed male Wistar rats. Am J Physiol Endocrin Metab 289:E1015–E1022, 2005b

Winsberg ME, DeGolia SG, Strong CM, et al: Divalproex therapy in medication-naive and mood-stabilizer-naive bipolar II depression. J Affect Disord 67:207–212, 2001

Yen DJ, Yu HY, Guo YC, et al: A double-blind, placebo-controlled study of topiramate in adult patients with refractory partial epilepsy. Epilepsia 41:1162–1166, 2000

Young LT, Robb JC, Hasey GM, et al: Gabapentin as an adjunctive treatment in bipolar disorder. J Affect Disord 55:73–77, 1999

Young LT, Joffe RT, Robb JC, et al: Double-blind comparison of addition of a second mood stabilizer versus an antidepressant to an initial mood stabilizer for treatment of patients with bipolar depression. Am J Psychiatry 157:124–126, 2000

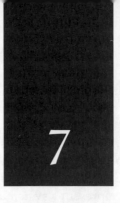

ANTIDEPRESSANTS IN BIPOLAR DEPRESSION

Rif S. El-Mallakh, M.D.
Anoop Karippot, M.D.
S. Nassir Ghaemi, M.D., M.P.H.

TREATMENT AND PREVENTION OF bipolar depression is a major problem in the long-term treatment of bipolar illness. While about one-third of patients may experience adequate prophylaxis with lithium or valproate (El-Mallakh 1994), the majority of patients continue to be symptomatic (Ghaemi 2002). For example, although gender distribution of the bipolar diagnosis is equal, women may experience depression at two or three times the rate in men (Goodwin and Jamison 1990). Additionally, depressive symptoms themselves may be more problematic: both type I and type II bipolar disorder patients spend one-third to half of their lives, respectively, experiencing depressive symptoms (Judd et al. 2002, 2003). This depressive morbidity is at least three times as common as manic or hypomanic morbidity (Ghaemi et al. 2000; Post et al. 2003a).

Early onset of depression appears to be an especially poor prognostic factor. Among 72 children who have experienced a prepubertal, major depressive episode followed for a mean of 10 years, 35 (48.6%) developed a bipolar disorder (mostly type I) (Geller et al. 2001). Therefore, it is thus not surprising that antidepressants are among the most frequently used class of drugs in bipolar illness (Ghaemi et al. 2000) and that their use in children can be especially problematic.

It would seem logical that the main class of agents used to treat bipolar depression should be antidepressants. Unfortunately, scientific evidence and clinical experience suggests that antidepressants are not the simple solution to the problem of bipolar depression.

This chapter does not represent a systematic review of the literature on antidepressants in bipolar depression. Such reviews have been published both for acute antidepressant effect (Gijsman et al. 2004) and for long-term prophylaxis (Ghaemi et al. 2001). In this chapter, while referring to those reviews, we will discuss the relevant randomized clinical trial (RCT) literature, as well as selected observational studies, so as to provide an interpretation of this literature. We seek here to digest this literature for the reader, not to be comprehensive and ask the reader to do the digestive activity. Thus, inevitably, there will be studies and viewpoints that will not be fully described here. Readers should see this chapter as an attempt to express our perspective on this complex field.

EFFICACY

The efficacy of antidepressants in bipolar depression should be considered in two phases, acute and maintenance, and further assessed in the different diagnostic subtypes of the illness.

Acute Efficacy in Bipolar I Disorder

In the acute phase, a good amount of evidence suggests that antidepressants are more effective than placebo (mostly in the absence of concomitant mood stabilizer) or that certain antidepressants may be more effective than others in RCTs of the acute major depressive episode in bipolar disorder (Amsterdam 1998; Amsterdam et al. 1998; Cohn et al. 1989; Himmelhoch et al. 1982, 1991; Simpson et al. 1991; Thase et al. 1992).

In a set of influential, double-blind, placebo-controlled, randomized studies of anergic depression, Himmelhoch et al. (1982, 1991) found that the monoamine oxidase inhibitors (MAOIs) were superior to imipramine in 56 depressed bipolar subjects (total number of subjects not reported). Similarly, another RCT (Thase et al.1992) reported that 9 out of 12 (75%) nonresponders to imipramine responded to tranylcypromine, whereas only 1 out of 4 (25%) nonresponders to the MAOI responded to imipramine.

Those early studies did not use concomitant mood stabilizers. In the only RCT to assess antidepressant efficacy in lithium-treated patients, imipramine and paroxetine were not overall more effective than placebo when added to lithium for treatment of the acute depressive symptoms in patients with bipolar disorder type I. However, in a secondary analysis of those with low lithium levels (<0.8), both antidepressants were superior to placebo when added to lithium (Nemeroff et al. 2001).

A more recent study performed to demonstrate the efficacy of the combination of olanzapine and fluoxetine in bipolar depression may shed light on the utility of fluoxetine. The study had an olanzapine-only arm, an olanzapine-plus-fluoxetine arm, and a placebo arm. Patients in both active arms improved. The effect size for the olanzapine-only arm was only 0.3, while the effect size of the combination was about 0.65 (Tohen et al. 2004). Although the authors argued that there may be a synergistic effect between the two drugs, the observed effect size of the combination is similar to fluoxetine alone in unipolar depression (e.g., Stark and Hardison 1985). Additionally, the issue of synergy cannot adequately be inferred from the study without a fluoxetine-only arm. Thus, this study suggests that fluoxetine alone may be more effective than nothing. Clinically meaningful efficacy of the olanzapine component of the study was not proven.

An earlier study of fluoxetine compared it with imipramine and placebo in a double-blind RCT (Cohn et al. 1989). However, this was a quite poorly designed study. About one-third of the patients received lithium, and the rest were taking no mood stabilizers. The published paper reports conflicting data on who received lithium; it appears that lithium may have been much more frequently used in the fluoxetine arm. If that is the case, then the study is a comparison of fluoxetine plus lithium versus imipramine alone, hardly a balanced comparison. Thus the success of randomization in this study is in doubt, and its results, which report better efficacy with fluoxetine (86%) compared with imipramine (57%), are best discounted.

In summary, some antidepressants may be more effective than others in treating bipolar depression. However, in an adequately designed RCT, no antidepressant has yet been shown to be more effective than lithium in the treatment of bipolar depression.

Acute Efficacy in Bipolar II Disorder

Some investigators suggest that antidepressants may be effective in type II bipolar depression. In a post hoc pooled analysis of unipolar RCTs, 89 bipolar II subjects were identified in a cohort of 839 fluoxetine-treated patients (Amsterdam et al. 1998; note that this was in the DSM-III-R era in which hypomania was not diagnosed). When these subjects were compared with either 89 age- and gender-matched unipolar patients or 661 unmatched unipolar subjects, it was found that the efficacy of fluoxetine was equal in the bipolar and unipolar groups. These results may not be valid because of the post hoc nature of the analysis (with inflated false-positive chance findings) and the pooled nature of the study (which results in loss of the benefit of randomization, due to reintroduction of clinical and demographic differences between studies that may influence the results).

A similar post hoc reanalysis of unipolar depression RCTs with venlafaxine was conducted by the same group (Amsterdam and Garcia-Espana 2000). The investigators identified 15 bipolar II women (mean age 37±12 years) whom they matched to 17 unipolar women (mean age 41±12 years). All women were depressed (baseline Ham-D 21-item score was 23.5) and followed for 6 weeks. Two bipolar (13%) and three unipolar (18%) women discontinued the study early. No one experienced hypomania as characterized by agitation, irritability, euphoria, or mood lability, but mania scales were not completed. By week 6 there were similar improvements in both unipolar women (Ham-D 11±7) and bipolar women (Ham-D 11±9) and similar response rates in both groups (defined as >50% improvement in Ham-D at 60% in unipolar and 63% in bipolar women). The same methodological critiques mentioned in the previous study discussed also apply to this analysis.

Recently, the same investigators (Amsterdam et al. 2004) openly administered fluoxetine monotherapy at a fixed dose of 20 mg/day to 37 depressed type II bipolar subjects. Twenty-three patients (62%) completed the 8-week study. Of these, 11 (48% of completers, 30% of intent to treat sample) responded with a reduction in Ham-D (17-item) scores of >50%. Young Mania Scale scores did not appreciably increase above baseline in the sample but three patients experienced hypomania (8.1%) and one stopped the study due to a rapid mood swing into a depression (Amsterdam et al. 2004). There was no placebo arm, so the switch rate of 8% could not be compared with the natural switch rate of this sample.

Finally, in an open-label, nonrandomized study, Amsterdam (1998) reported 6 weeks of venlafaxine (225 mg/day) monotherapy in 17 type II depressed subjects. Reduction in both the 21-item Ham-D (22.0±6.0 to 9.0±7.0) and the Montgomery-Åsberg Depression Rating Scale (MADRS) (22.0±7.0 to 9.0±8.0) was significant and equivalent to that seen in 26 unipolar subjects.

None of these studies represent the kind of study that is needed to prove efficacy of antidepressants in type II bipolar depression, namely a prospective, double-blind, RCT of sufficient size. No such study has been conducted with standard antidepressants. Therefore, while one might conclude based on the above studies that such efficacy might exist, better research is needed to prove it.

The conclusions just discussed may seem to conflict with a recent meta-analysis of RCTs of antidepressants for bipolar depression (Gijsman et al. 2004), which concluded that short-term antidepressants are effective in bipolar depression and that overall switch rates into mania/hypomania appear similar for antidepressants (3.8%) and placebo (4.7%). Yet there are major problems with the validity of this meta-analysis (Ghaemi and Goodwin 2005). Methodologically, meta-analyses represent an observational study of studies; even if the component studies are randomized, the meta-analytic result is not randomized (Colditz et al. 1995). Thus it is liable to confounding bias—that is, the possibility that factors other than the presumed cause (e.g., antidepressant use) may differ among the studies and thereby account for an observed result. This potential for heterogeneity requires statistical exploration, and although it does not invalidate meta-analysis findings, it does (as with any observational study) require readers to critically assess results.

Only four placebo-controlled studies in the meta-analysis by Gijsman et al. (2004) met their criteria and provided the data needed to assess acute antidepressant efficacy. Two were studies from the early 1980s that used no concomitant mood stabilizers. The third study utilized fluoxetine but equivocated on whether it equally allocated patients to baseline lithium treatment; the fluoxetine group appeared to receive lithium more frequently than did the imipramine group, creating an unbalanced comparison. The fourth study, contributing a disproportionate majority of subjects to this meta-analysis, compared olanzapine with olanzapine plus fluoxetine—thus, the "placebo" group in that study was actually olanzapine. The sum of these differences in study design, alongside differences in patient characteristics across studies, throw doubt onto whether the overall results of the meta-analysis are accurate. Sources of heterogeneity across individual studies require that the meta-analysis findings be interpreted with great caution.

Moreover, the aggregate of these studies has not clarified the fundamental controversy over whether or not it is effective to add an antidepressant to a therapeutic dose of a proven mood stabilizer. This has been adequately addressed in only one study, Nemeroff et al. (2001), which found that adding either a selective serotonin reuptake inhibitor or tricyclic antidepressant was not more effective than using therapeutically dosed lithium. A second, preliminary, randomized trial found similar antidepressant responses in depressed bipolar patients who took lithium plus divalproex versus each of these plus paroxetine (Gijsman et al. 2004).

In sum, the heterogeneity across controlled studies incurs a risk for drawing oversimplistic generalizations about presumed efficacy or safety without attention to the problem of confounding biases in study design.

Prophylactic Efficacy in Bipolar Disorder

All of the above discussion only relates to acute efficacy. What should one do when the patient is *currently* depressed? If one uses an antidepressant, the next question is what should be done after recovery from the current depression. If the patient responds to an antidepressant, should it be continued or not? In other words, do antidepressants prevent new depressive episodes in bipolar disorder?

The available evidence suggests that, overall, antidepressants do not appear to have long-term preventive benefits in bipolar depression. There have been six double-blind RCTs of prophylaxis of bipolar disorder with antidepressants (Ghaemi et al. 2003). Those studies all compared imipramine with placebo or with lithium. In all cases, imipramine alone or with the addition of lithium were not more effective than lithium alone in the prevention of mood episodes in bipolar disorder. In all cases, there was no added benefit from using imipramine long term. Thus, if one were to conduct a systematic review of the RCT literature on antidepressants in prophylaxis of bipolar disorder (as has been done by Ghaemi et al. 2001), one would have to conclude, in contrast to the above meta-analysis of the acute treatment literature, that antidepressants are not effective in the prophylaxis of bipolar disorder.

This literature has been criticized on two grounds. First, some studies did not assess prophylaxis in those who had recovered with imipramine for the acute major depressive episode. Second, the studies utilized imipramine, a tricyclic antidepressant (TCA); the results might be more favorable for newer antidepressants, such as serotonin reuptake inhibitors (SRIs).

To address these two issues, we now have two new, as yet unpublished RCTs. In the first (Post et al. 2004), venlafaxine was compared with bupropion and sertraline when added to standard mood stabilizers. In the overall results, similar numbers of patients experienced acute response (53.2%–59.7%), but there was more manic switch with venlafaxine (15.1% vs. 5.4% for bupropion and 6.7% with sertraline). Remission without any manic switch at 1 year was only seen in 17.9% of patients with venlafaxine, 27.4% with sertraline, and 38.1% with bupropion.

In a second ongoing RCT (in process by our group; Ghaemi et al. 2005), patients were studied after initial recovery with a mood stabilizer plus an antidepressant for acute bipolar depression. Responders were then openly randomized to continue or discontinue antidepressant (while staying on a mood stabilizer). Interim analysis of 66 patients suggests no added benefit to remaining on antidepressant for long-term treatment. In a planned, subgroup analysis, patients with rapid-cycling bipolar disorder had more depressive morbidity in the 1-year follow-up when continuing antidepressants as opposed to discontinuing antidepressants.

These studies suggest that antidepressants are not effective when added to mood stabilizers in the long-term prevention of mood episodes in bipolar disorder in which most patients have type I disorder.

Patients with type II or not otherwise specified (NOS) bipolar disorder may benefit from prolonged antidepressant treatment. Amsterdam and Shults (2005) performed a double-blind, placebo-substitution, continuation study in which patients responding to open treatment with fluoxetine 20 mg (defined as achieving euthymia with a Ham-D score of ≤9) were randomized to placebo or fluoxetine 20 g/day for 6 months. All of the placebo-treated patients relapsed, whereas only 43% of the fluoxetine-treated patients relapsed. Because of the small sample size of the study, this difference did not reach statistical difference ($P=0.08$). However, the Young Mania Scale score significantly increased in the fluoxetine-treated subjects (3.0 ± 1.8 vs. 0.2 ± 0.4 points, $P=0.01$) versus the placebo-treated patients (Amsterdam and Shults 2005). These results suggest a small depressive prophylactic effect and a significant pro-hypomanic effect in type II and NOS bipolar patients receiving fluoxetine.

SAFETY

The safety of antidepressants in bipolar depression should be considered for two phases: acute and long-term depression (mood destabilization and/or rapid cycling) and further assessed in the different diagnostic subtypes of the illness.

Antidepressant-Induced Acute Mania

Does acute mania occur with antidepressant treatment, and if so, how frequent does it? To assess whether it occurs, one would ideally need

RCTs designed to answer the question. However, RCTs of antidepressants in bipolar depression are not designed to assess side effects like acute mania induction; rather, they are designed to assess efficacy. This leads to the common mistake of saying that there is no risk for a side effect like mania induction because of the lack of statistical significance for such risk. However, absence of evidence is not evidence of absence—such studies would need to include about 10,000 patients to demonstrate statistical differences between antidepressant and placebo, given the low rates seen in RCTs.

The rates of acute mania seen in RCTs of acute bipolar depression tend to hover around 5% for placebo, compared with 0%–50% for antidepressants, depending on the study. The overall numbers tend to be lower than reported in observational studies. A possible reason for the lower rates is that patients who enter RCTs are a highly selected population: these persons typically are not severely ill, do not have psychiatric or medical comorbidities, and are highly compliant and motivated. Such persons may not possess some of the risk factors for antidepressant-induced mania (such as substance abuse comorbidity). Therefore, one should not place great emphasis on the actual frequency of acute mania seen in RCTs because this is likely an underestimate of the frequency in the real world. Furthermore, one should not pay attention to statistical significance (or P values) because such RCTs are woefully underpowered to assess acute mania. The main question is whether, given the limitations of the RCT design, antidepressants cause acute mania more frequently than placebo does.

Regarding antidepressant-induced mania, the meta-analysis described above reported no such risk (Gijsman et al. 2004). However, 58% of the subjects in this meta-analysis were derived from only one study that involved an olanzapine-fluoxetine combination (OFC), which single-handedly drove the results. Since "placebo" in the analysis was actually olanzapine or placebo, one can conclude only that antidepressants may not cause mania in the setting of antimanic agents. Two studies reported no mania at all, with placebo or antidepressant, suggesting possible measurement bias (inadequate assessment of manic symptoms). Another found an unfavorable relative risk of manic switch with imipramine versus paroxetine, but the two groups were combined for the meta-analysis, thus washing away the likely tricyclic-related increased risk. In that study, Nemeroff et al. (2001) found that switch into mania occurred more frequently at lithium levels less than 0.8 mEq/L. At these lower levels, 11% of imipramine-treated subjects and 5% of mood-stabilizer alone–treated subjects (spontaneous rate) became manic or hypomanic. At lithium levels greater than 0.8 mEq/L, none of the mood-stabilizer-alone subjects switched, whereas 8% of the imipramine-treated subjects experienced a switch. None of the 33 paroxetine-treated subjects experienced a switch into mania or hypomania (Nemeroff et al. 2001).

Thus, the available placebo-controlled RCTs do not shed much light on the question of which method of treatment is more likely to induce mania one way or the other, with the exception that TCAs appear to have a higher risk than other antidepressants.

How common is antidepressant-induced mania in the real world? To answer this question, one needs to look at well-designed observational studies. In fact, observational studies are often more useful than RCTs in identifying safety risks in medications. A number of studies have been conducted, but one of the best designed, in terms of prospective assessment of this issue with mood rating scales, found about a 20%–25% manic switch rate with SRIs, which was similar to TCAs in this study (Henry et al. 2001). Other studies have reported somewhat higher rates with TCAs, in the 30%–60% range (Goodwin and Jamison 1990). In another observational study, about 50% of patients with bipolar disorder experienced antidepressant-induced acute mania at some point in their lives (Ghaemi et al. 2004). Thus, it is likely that 20%–60% of persons with bipolar disorder type I will develop antidepressant-induced acute mania at least once and even more frequently with TCAs than SRIs. Frequency of antidepressant-induced mania in bipolar disorder type II may be lower, although this topic has not been carefully studied.

The rate of antidepressant-induced mania in unipolar depression, in contrast, is much smaller than in bipolar disorder. For instance, in the study by Amsterdam et al. (1998), the manic switch rate in bipolar II disorder, though low, was four times higher than in unipolar depression (4% vs. 1%). Other observational studies tend to report no or very little antidepressant-induced mania in those for whom unipolar depression was appropriately diagnosed (Ghaemi et al. 2004).

Risk Factors for Antidepressant-Induced Acute Mania

Although definitive risk factors are not established, a number of studies suggest some likely factors for antidepressant-induced mania (Goldberg and Truman 2003). Antidepressant-induced manias have a significant irritability component, often resembling mixed rather than pure manic episodes (Stoll et al. 1994). This feature may be an important component of the potential for increased suicidality in some persons treated with antidepressants, because mixed episodes are associated with elevated suicidality (Dilsaver et al. 1994). Additionally, subjects with cyclothymia may convert to a type II illness when given antidepressants (Akiskal et al. 1977). Hyperthymic personality (a chronic baseline hypomanic state) appears to increase the risk of antidepressant-induced mania (Henry et al. 2001). Importantly, current or past substance abuse appears to be a major predictor of antidepressant-induced manic switch (Goldberg and Whiteside 2002; Manwani et al. 2005). Young age may also be a risk factor. In one study (Biederman et al. 2000), the SRIs were associated with a high probability of inducing manic symptoms (hazards ratio=3.0 [1.2–7.8], $P=0.02$).

The mood state of the individual when he or she is given antidepressants may be an important determinant in the induction of mania. El-Mallakh (2001) reported a case of type I bipolar patient whose depression improved with the addition of bupropion without any adverse consequence, but who developed a mania when he took the same medication for smoking cessation while euthymic.

Lastly, treatment with antidepressant monotherapy, in the absence of a mood stabilizer, likely increases the risk of induction of acute mania (Ghaemi et al. 2004). This is most likely to occur in the setting of the misdiagnosis of bipolar disorder as unipolar depression, which has been shown to occur in about 40% of persons with bipolar disorder (Hirschfeld et al. 2003). Due to misdiagnosis, there is a frequent delay of over 5 years for the diagnosis of type I illness and over a decade for the diagnosis of a type II illness after the initial contact is made with a mental health practitioner; by the time of correct bipolar diagnosis, 78% have already been prescribed antidepressants, often in monotherapy (Ghaemi et al. 2000).

Antidepressant-Induced Mood Destabilization and/or Rapid Cycling

Whether antidepressants can destabilize mood in the long run has been controversial. The best evidence for such an effect comes from three RCTs. In the first study, manic episodes were reported almost 2.5 times more frequently in bipolar type I patients with double-blind treatment of lithium plus imipramine (24%) compared with lithium alone (10%) over a mean 1.6-year follow-up (Quitkin et al. 1986). These results were statistically significant in the female subgroup. Depressive relapse rates were similar for lithium alone (10%) compared with lithium plus imipramine.

The second study, a small, placebo-controlled, on-off-on design

RCT, also demonstrated a pattern of increased cycling with TCAs (Wehr and Goodwin 1979). This study reported that time between affective switches was almost four times shorter with desipramine compared with lithium monotherapy.

The third controlled study assessed 51 rapid-cycling patients who were admitted to the National Institute of Mental Health (NIMH) over a 10-year period (Wehr et al. 1988). Nonrandomized assessments of treatment response history suggested antidepressants were associated with rapid cycling in 51% of patients. After prospective, double-blind, randomized replacement of antidepressant with placebo, the study concluded that 33% (17/51) experienced rapid cycling directly related to antidepressants. Wehr and colleagues further studied that subgroup of 17 patients more intensely, and determined, through repeated on-off-on-off design, that antidepressant use was definitively associated with rapid cycling in 10 patients from the original sample (19.6%). Thus, this study, which probably represents the most rigorous examination of this issue, demonstrates with high likelihood a causative association between antidepressants and rapid cycling that can be conservatively estimated at about 20%, at least in a highly refractory population such as that seen at the NIMH.

It is sometimes asserted that since other RCTs have not found evidence of worsened outcomes with antidepressants (they found no improvement but also no worsening), we can conclude that antidepressants may not cause such outcomes. Again, it is important always to keep in mind that the only study designed to directly address this issue (Wehr et al. 1988) did find evidence of antidepressant use leading to rapid-cycling course. Other RCTs were not designed to assess the issue, did not have sufficient power to find it, and did not assess subgroups that might be at special risk, such as those with rapid cycling illness. Again, absence of evidence is not evidence of absence. Despite all the reasons why such poor outcomes might be missed, it is worrisome that one of those RCTs (Quitkin et al. 1981) still found such evidence.

Observational Studies

If one is convinced, based on the above RCT evidence, that antidepressant-induced rapid-cycling or mood destabilization can occur, he or she can then turn to the observational literature to look at clinical nuances of this association.

In the pre-antidepressant era (pre-1950s), rapid cycling among bipolar subjects was quite rare (Kukopulos et al. 1983). Since then, several studies have reported an association. In one report, the cycling terminated when antidepressants were discontinued in about one-third of patients (Wehr et al. 1988). In a retrospective chart review of 109 rapid-cycling bipolar patients, Kukopulos et al. (1983) found that 80 (73.4%) developed rapid cycling some time after onset of bipolar illness. Specifically, 65 type II and 15 type I individuals developed rapid cycling 11 years after the onset of the bipolar disorder. The number of episodes per year grew from 0.8 to 6.5. In all 80 subjects, onset of rapid cycling was associated with antidepressant treatment that continued through euthymic periods ($n=17$) or that persisted at least 1 year ($n=33$), 2 years ($n=14$), or longer ($n=5$). The authors pointed out that since 52 of these patients had depressive episodes prior to antidepressant exposure (and were treated with psychotherapy, anxiolytics, electroconvulsive therapy [ECT], or not at all), the occurrence of depression, per se, was not the precipitant of rapid cycling. Their conclusion was that antidepressants may be responsible for the apparent increase in the prevalence of rapid cycling.

Altshuler et al. (1995) reviewed the life charts of 51 patients with treatment refractory bipolar illness. Although retrospective, the technique allowed them to identify antidepressant-associated mania or cycle acceleration. They found that 35% of patients had antidepressant-associated manic episodes and 26% experienced cycle acceleration. Antidepressant-induced mania was associated with increased risk of cycle acceleration (46% vs. 14% in subjects without antidepressant-induced mania). Additionally, younger age at first treatment predicted cycle acceleration. Because antidepressant treatment is more likely to precede mood stabilizer treatment (Ghaemi et al. 2000), that prolonged antidepressant exposure may increase vulnerability. However, this was not assessed in the study (Altshuler et al. 1995).

Ghaemi et al. (2000) reviewed the charts of 54 bipolar subjects (27 type I, 11 type II, and 16 not otherwise specified) who received diagnosis by a modified, structured, clinical interview for diagnosis (SCID, DSM-IV criteria). Forty-two subjects had received antidepressant treatment at some point and, of these, only 38 had sufficient data for analysis. Fifty-five percent developed mania or hypomania and 23% experienced cycle acceleration. Interestingly, while the number of annual episodes increased from an average of 3.9 to 9.8 ($Z=-1.29$, $P=0.02$, $n=16$), the episodes were sufficiently brief that absolute amount of time spent ill dropped from 60% to 45% ($Z=-1.80$, $P=0.07$, $n=16$) (Ghaemi et al. 2000).

Rapid cycling faded quickly in 15 of 51 subjects (29%) studied by Wehr et al. (1988). Similarly, 8 of 9 subjects (89%) studied by Altshuler et al. (1995) experienced discontinuation of rapid cycling within 2 months of stopping the antidepressant. However, one patient cycled for 5 months prior to stabilizing after antidepressant discontinuation (Altshuler et al. 1995).

ANTIDEPRESSANT-ASSOCIATED CHRONIC IRRITABLE DYSPHORIA

In 1987, Akiskal and Mallya introduced the notion of antidepressant-induced, chronic symptoms that include irritability and sleep disturbance in relatives of bipolar patients who have only manifested unipolar depressions. These patients developed a syndrome that consists of 1) unrelenting dysphoria, 2) severe agitation, 3) refractory anxiety, 4) unendurable sexual excitement, 5) intractable insomnia, 6) suicidal obsessions and impulses, and 7) "histrionic demeanor" (Akiskal and Mallya 1987). More recently, El-Mallakh and Karippot (2005) have described a chronic irritable depressive state that develops after long-term (several years) treatment with antidepressants in both type I and type II patients. This syndrome is specifically manifested by a triad of dysphoria, middle insomnia, and irritability, and thus has been labeled antidepressant-associated chronic irritable dysphoria (ACID). Patients with ACID invariably experience significant social and occupational dysfunction such as divorce, separation, and disability. Discontinuation of the antidepressants usually results in improvement of all ACID symptoms and a return of both social and occupational function within about 6–8 months of not taking antidepressants. In 83 subjects studied in the Systematic Treatment Enhancement Program for Bipolar Disorder (STEP-BD) study who developed a depression after entering the study, those receiving antidepressants were more likely to develop ACID than those not receiving an antidepressant (R.S. El-Mallakh, S.N. Ghaemi, K. Sagduyu, et al., "Antidepressant-associated chronic irritable dysphoria [ACID] in STEP-BD patients," University of Louisville, 2005). Additional work is required to investigate this syndrome.

SUMMARY

In summary, the available evidence seems to suggest the following: regarding efficacy, antidepressants appear to be effective in the acute major depressive episode compared with no treatment, but they appear to be equivalent to lithium monotherapy at therapeutic levels. For long-term prophylaxis, antidepressants do not appear to be effective overall. However, a subgroup of perhaps 15%–40% of patients may benefit from long-term antidepressant treatment.

Regarding safety, antidepressants appear to cause acute manic episodes in about 20%–50% of individuals with bipolar disorder, perhaps more so in type I than type II. Long-term antidepressants cause mood destabilization and worsening of the course of bipolar illness in about 25%–40% of persons with bipolar disorder.

Antidepressants can have a role in the treatment of bipolar disorder, but special caution needs to be used to find that minority of patients in whom antidepressants can be helpful, and to avoid that minority in whom they can be harmful. At the same time, widespread use of these agents in long-term treatment appears to be unjustified because of their lack of prophylactic efficacy.

REFERENCES

Akiskal HS, Djenderedjian AT, Rosenthal RH, et al: Cyclothymic disorder: validating criteria for inclusion in the bipolar affective group. Am J Psychiatry 134:1227–1233, 1977

Akiskal HS, Mallya G: Criteria for the "soft" bipolar spectrum: treatment implications. Psychopharmacol Bull 23:68–73, 1987

Altshuler LL, Post RM, Leverich GS, et al: Antidepressant-induced mania and cycle acceleration: a controversy revisited. Am J Psychiatry 152:1130–1138, 1995

Amsterdam J: Efficacy and safety of venlafaxine in treatment of bipolar II major depressive episode. J Clin Psychopharmacol 18:414–417, 1998

Amsterdam JD, Garcia-Espana F: Venlafaxine monotherapy in women with bipolar II and unipolar major depression. J Affect Disord 59:225–229, 2000

Amsterdam JD, Shults J: Flouxetine monotherapy of bipolar type II and bipolar NOS major depression: a double-blind, placebo-substitution, continuation study. Int Clin Psychopharmacol 20:257–264, 2005

Amsterdam JD, Garcia-Espana F, Fawcett J, et al: Efficacy and safety of fluoxetine in treating bipolar II major depressive episode. J Clin Psychopharmacol 18:435–440, 1998

Amsterdam JD, Shults J, Brunswick DJ, Hundert M: Short-term fluoxetine monotherapy for bipolar type II or bipolar NOS major depression—low manic switch rate. Bipolar Disord 6:75–81, 2004

Biederman J, Mick E, Spencer TJ, et al.: Therapeutic dilemmas in the pharmacotherapy of bipolar depression in the young. J Child Adolesc Psychopharmacol 10:185–192, 2000

Cohn JB, Collins G, Ashbrook E, et al: A comparison of fluoxetine, imipramine and placebo in patients with bipolar depressive disorder. Int Clin Psychopharmacol 4:313–322, 1989

Colditz GA, Burdick E, Mosteller F: Heterogeneity in meta-analysis of data from epidemiologic studies: a commentary: Am J Epidemiol 142:371–382, 1995

Dilsaver S, Chen Y, Swann A, et al: Suicidality in patients with pure and depressive mania. Am J Psychiatry 151: 1312–1315, 1994

EI-Mallakh RS: Lithium: Actions and Mechanisms. Washington, DC, American Psychiatric Press, 1994

El-Mallakh RS: Bupropion manic induction during euthymia but not during depression. Bipolar Disord 3:159–160, 2001

El-Mallakh RS, Karippot A: Antidepressant-associated chronic irritable dysphoria (ACID) in bipolar disorder. J Affect Disord 84:267–272, 2005

Geller B, Zimerman B, Williams M, et al: Bipolar disorder at prospective follow-up of adults who had prepubertal major depressive disorder. Am J Psychiatry 158: 125–127, 2001

Ghaemi SN (ed): Polypharmacy in Psychiatry. New York, Marcel Dekker, 2002

Ghaemi SN, Goodwin FK: Antidepressants for bipolar depression. Am J Psychiatry 162:1545–1546, 2005

Ghaemi SN, Boiman EE, Goodwin FK: Diagnosing bipolar disorder and the effect of antidepressants: a naturalistic study. J Clin Psychiatry 61:804–808, 2000

Ghaemi SN, Lenox MS, Baldessarini RJ: Effectiveness and safety of long-term antidepressant treatment in bipolar disorder. J Clin Psychiatry 62:565–569, 2001

Ghaemi SN, Hsu DJ, Soldani F, et al: Antidepressants in bipolar disorder: the case for caution. Bipolar Disord 5:421–433, 2003

Ghaemi SN, Rosenquist KJ, Ko JY, et al: Antidepressant treatment in bipolar versus unipolar depression. Am J Psychiatry 161:163–165, 2004

Ghaemi SN, El-Mallakh RS, Baldassano CF, et al: A randomized clinical trial of efficacy and safety of long-term antidepressant use in bipolar disorder (abstract). Bipolar Disord 7 (suppl 2):59, 2005

Gijsman HJ, Geddes JR, Rendell JM, et al: Antidepressants for bipolar depression: a systematic review of randomized, controlled trials. Am J Psychiatry 161:1537–1547, 2004

Goldberg J, Whiteside J: The association between substance abuse and antidepressant-induced mania in bipolar disorder: a preliminary study. J Clin Psychiatry 63:791–795, 2002

Goldberg JF, Truman CJ: Antidepressant-induced mania: an overview of current controversies. Bipolar Disord 5:407–420, 2003

Goodwin F, Jamison K: Manic Depressive Illness. New York, Oxford University Press, 1990

Henry C, Sorbara F, Lacoste J, et al: Antidepressant-induced mania in bipolar patients: identification of risk factors: J Clin Psychiatry 62:249–255, 2001

Himmelhoch JM, Fuchs CZ, Symons BJ: A double-blind study of tranylcypro-mine treatment of major anergic depression. J Nerv Mental Disease 170:628–634, 1982

Himmelhoch JM, Thase ME, Mallinger AG, et al: Tranylcypromine versus imi-pramine in anergic bipolar depression. Am J Psychiatry 148:910–916, 1991

Hirschfeld RM, Lewis L, Vornik LA: Perceptions and impact of bipolar disorder: how far have we really come? Results of the national depressive and manic-depressive association 2000 survey of individuals with bipolar dis-order. J Clin Psychiatry 64:161–174, 2003

Judd LL, Akiskal HS, Schettler PJ, et al: The long-term natural history of the weekly symptomatic status of bipolar I disorder. Arch Gen Psychiatry 59:530–537, 2002

Judd LL, Akiskal HS, Schettler PJ, et al: A prospective investigation of the nat-ural history of the long-term weekly symptomatic status of bipolar II dis-order. Arch Gen Psychiatry 60:261–269, 2003

Kukopulos A, Caliari B, Tundi A, et al: Rapid cyclers, temperament, and antide-pressants. Comprehen Psychiatry 24:249–258, 1983

Manwani S, Pardo TB, Albanese M, et al: Bipolar disorder, substance abuse, and antidepressant induced mania (abstract). Bipolar Disord 7 (suppl 2):75, 2005

Nemeroff CB, Evans DL, Gyulai L, et al: A double-blind, placebo-controlled comparison of imipramine and paroxetine in the treatment of bipolar de-pression. Am J Psychiatry 158:906–912, 2001

Post RM, Denicoff KD, Leverich GS, et al: Morbidity in 258 bipolar outpatients followed for 1 year with daily prospective ratings on the NIMH life chart method. J Clin Psychiatry 64:680–690, 2003a

Post R, Altshuler L, Leverich G, et al: Randomized comparison of bupropion, sertraline, and venlafaxine as adjunctive treatment in acute bipolar depres-sion, in New Research and Abstracts, 157th Annual Meeting of the Ameri-can Psychiatric Association. New York, May 1–6, 2004. Washington DC, American Psychiatric Association, 2004, pp 259–265

Quitkin FM, Kane J, Rifkin A, et al: Prophylactic lithium carbonate with and without imipramine for bipolar I patients: a double-blind study. Arch Gen Psychiatry 38:902–907, 1981

Quitkin FM, Rabkin JG , Stewart JW, et al: Study duration in antidepressant re-search: advantages of a 12-week trial. J Psychiatr Res 20:211–216, 1986

Sachs GS, Printz DJ, Kahn DA, et al: The Expert Consensus Guidelines Series: medication treatment of bipolar disorder 2000. Postgrad Med April:1–104, 2000

Simpson SG, DePaulo JR: Fluoxetine treatment for bipolar II depression. J Clin Psychopharmacol 11:52–54, 1991

Stark P, Hardison CD: A review of multicenter controlled studies of fluoxetine vs imipramine and placebo in outpatients with major depressive disorder. J Clin Psychiatry 46:53–58, 1985

Stoll AL, Mayer PB, Kolbrener M, et al: Antidepressant-associated mania: a controlled comparison with spontaneous mania. Am J Psychiatry 151:1642–1645, 1994

Thase ME, Mallinger AG, McKnight D, et al: Treatment of imipramine-resistant recurrent depression. III: efficacy of monamine oxidase inhibitors. J Clin Psychiatry 53:5–11, 1992

Tohen M, Vieta E, Ketter T, et al: Efficacy of olanzapine and olanzapine-fluoxetine combination in the treatment of bipolar I depression. Arch Gen Psychiatry 60:1079–1088, 2003; erratum 61:176, 2004

Wehr T, Goodwin F: Rapid cycling in manic-depressives induced by tricyclic antidepressants. Arch Gen Psychiatry 36:555–559, 1979

Wehr TA, Sack DA, Rosenthal NE, et al: Rapid cycling affective disorder: contributing factors and treatment response in 51 patients. Am J Psychiatry 145:179–184, 1988

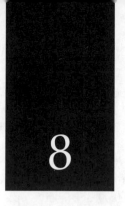

ANTIPSYCHOTICS IN BIPOLAR DEPRESSION

Rif S. El-Mallakh, M.D.

ANTIPSYCHOTICS ARE AMONG the most frequently used medications in bipolar illness. In studies of bipolar patients discharged from the hospital, 47%–90% of patients are prescribed antipsychotics alone or in combination with mood stabilizers (Keck et al. 1996; Tohen et al. 2001). Antipsychotics are continued in the outpatient setting for 60%–89% of patients for 6 months or longer (Keck et al. 1996; Ozerdem et al. 2001; Verdoux et al. 1996).

Until the introduction of the newer, second-generation antipsychotic medications, it was believed that antipsychotics did not play a significant therapeutic role in bipolar depression because first-generation antipsychotics had always been believed to produce depression or a depressive-like clinical picture.

ANTIPSYCHOTICS AS PRO-DEPRESSANTS

The depressogenic effect of first-generation antipsychotics is most evident in long-term, relapse-prevention studies. Ahlfors et al. (1981) reported a study of 93 patients who were switched to flupenthixol decanoate from lithium treatment due to inadequate prophylaxis (*n*=66), poor compliance (*n*=33), troublesome side effects (*n*=70), or fear of side effects

(n=22). Only 85 were bipolar, the remainder were unipolar depressives. Prospective data (over 14 months) were compared with patient retrospective illness over the 2 years prior to study entry. Flupenthixol was used because it had been previously reported to have an antidepressant effect in unipolar illness (Gruber and Cole 1991; Poldinger and Sieberns 1983). Despite this, patients experienced an increase in the number of depressive episodes (0.72 ± 0.09 depressive episodes/year on flupenthixol vs. 0.47 ± 0.07 depressive episodes/year prestudy, $P<0.05$). There was a significant reduction in manic episodes in the 85 bipolar subjects ($0.26\pm$SEM 0.06 manic episodes/year during study vs. 0.47 ± 0.07 manic episodes/year prestudy, $P<0.01$), but because depressions tend to last longer, the percentage of time spent ill with depression increased significantly ($12\pm2\%$ prestudy compared with $20\pm3\%$ on flupenthixol [$P<0.05$, Wilcoxon's matched pairs]), and the percentage of time spent ill with either mania or depression ($21\pm2\%$ prestudy vs. $26\pm3\%$ during study) was nonsignificantly increased (29%). The total number of episodes (0.95 ± 0.10 episodes/year prestudy vs. 0.97 ± 0.10 episodes/year during study) was not significantly different.

Similarly, White et al. (1993) performed a mirror-design study of depot antipsychotics in 16 patients with bipolar illness experiencing inadequate response to lithium or carbamazepine. When placed on haloperidol decanoate and followed prospectively for 44.4 months, these subjects experienced a significant decrease in manic episodes compared with the retrospectively investigated 44.4 months prior to the depot antipsychotic (from 1.25 ± 0.81 episodes/year prior to depot haloperidol to 0.51 ± 0.6 episodes/year on haloperidol decanoate, $P<0.01$), as well as a decrease in the percentage of time spent manic (from $15.4\%\pm11.8$ to $7.0\%\pm10.6$, $P<0.01$). There was a nonsignificant increase in the number of depressive episodes (from 0.12 ± 0.25 episodes/year to 0.15 ± 0.21 episodes/year, ns), and the percentage of time spent depressed (from $2.8\%\pm6.7$ to $4.7\%\pm10.3$, ns).

In a 6-month study of 37 bipolar patients stabilized from a manic episode using a mood stabilizer (lithium, valproate, or carbamazepine) plus perphenazine, subjects were randomly assigned to continue perphenazine or have it replaced by placebo (Zarate and Tohen 2004). Patients continuing perphenazine were more likely to relapse into depression or experience subsyndromal depressive symptoms or dysphoria compared with those receiving a mood stabilizer alone (Zarate and Tohen 2004).

By contrast, Littlejohn et al. (1994) reviewed the records of 18 bipolar subjects receiving depot neuroleptics with usable data. Mean duration of time spent off depot was 8.2 years (although they may have received oral antipsychotics) and time spent on depot was 6.3 years. Depot neuroleptics were associated with fewer hospitalizations (0.2 vs. 1.2 hospitalizations/year, $P < 0.001$), a reduction in the amount of time spent in the hospital (from 11.4 weeks/year to 1.5 weeks/year, $P < 0.001$), and fewer number of manic (1.0 vs. 9.1, $P < 0.001$), mixed (0 vs 1.0, $P < 0.01$), and depressive episodes (0.2 vs. 1.4, $P < 0.5$).

In addition to the effect of first-generation antipsychotics on depressive episodes, they are generally perceived as contributing to a depressive-like clinical picture. Most first-generation agents have potent dopamine D_2 receptor blockade. This results in amotivation, anhedonia, and bradykinesis, all of which look like depression even if the patient does not meet syndromal criteria for a major depressive episode.

ANTIPSYCHOTICS AS ANTIDEPRESSANTS

The introduction of the second generation of antipsychotics, with relatively less D_2 blockade and significant serotonin 5-HT_{2A} receptor blockade, suggested that these agents may be effective in bipolar illness without a significant depressogenic effect. This was insinuated in several short-term, placebo-controlled studies of second-generation antipsychotics in acute mania (Keck et al. 2003a, 2003b; Sachs et al. 2002; Tohen et al. 1999, 2000). In all of these studies, depressive scales were measured. All showed reductions in depressive symptoms in manic or mixed bipolar patients. However, depressive symptoms in mania are not depression, and the issue of whether these agents are antidepressive would have to be investigated in randomized trials of depressed bipolar subjects.

Olanzapine has been the most extensively studied agent in depressed bipolar subjects. In a double-blind, placebo-controlled study of nearly 750 depressed bipolar I patients, olanzapine monotherapy produced a statistically significant reduction compared with placebo in the Montgomery-Åsberg Depression Rating Scale (MADRS) (Tohen et al. 2003). However, the difference from placebo was only three points and was accounted for predominantly by improvements in sleep and appetite (Tohen et al. 2003), suggesting that the observed statistical difference was due to the side effects of olanzapine (sedation and increased appetite) and reached statistical significance due to the very large sample size. More important is the observation that over the 4 weeks of the study, olanzapine did not worsen the depression.

It has been suggested that when olanzapine is combined with fluoxetine there is a synergistic interaction that is uniquely antidepressive in bipolar illness (a notion that is reinforced by the name of the product, Symbiax). The United States Food and Drug Administration has recently approved this combination for acute bipolar depression based on a single, placebo-controlled study (Tohen et al. 2003). While it is clear that the olanzapine-fluoxetine combination (OFC) had a significant antidepressive effect, the observed effect size is not different that that observed for an SRI alone in unipolar depression (e.g., Stark and Hardison 1985). Nonetheless, the combination may indeed reduce manic induction that may occur with fluoxetine if given alone (Tohen et al. 2003).

Long-term studies with the OFC have been done but have not been presented nor published. However, long-term administration of olanzapine has been investigated. Olanzapine added to lithium or valproate after a patient has recovered with lithium or valproate monotherapy delayed symptomatic but not syndromal relapse over 18 months compared with mood stabilizer alone (Tohen et al. 2004).

Quetiapine was also investigated in a double-blind, placebo-controlled study in bipolar depression (Calabrese et al. 2005). This study also examined a large number of depressed bipolar subjects ($N=542$ of which 360 were type I and 182 were type II). Over the course of the 8-week study, quetiapine at either 300 mg/day or 600 mg/day significantly reduced both MADRS and Hamilton Rating Scale for Depression (17-item) score. The effect size of approximately 0.67 for 300 mg and 0.81 for 600 mg difference from placebo is mildly better than generally seen with antidepressant agents. An analysis of the MADRS items found that all items (except appetite) improved compared with placebo. Long-term effects have not been studied.

In an open, 6-month study of type II bipolar patients in which 14 patients received risperidone monotherapy and 30 patients received risperidone in combination with mood stabilizer, risperidone was associated with a very low rate of hypomania (4%, two patients had two episodes) and a seemingly low rate of depressive relapse (12%, nine patients had one episode each) (Vieta et al. 2001).

SUMMARY

There appears to be a real difference between the first- and second-generation antipsychotic medications. First-generation agents appear to increase both depressive episodes and depressive syndromes in bipolar patients receiving these drugs over the long term. Second-generation agents are either benign or actually reduce both acute and long-term depressive symptoms and syndromes. It appears unlikely that these agents will be adequate in controlling acute depressions and preventing depressive relapses in monotherapy. This effect appears to be true for olanzapine and quetiapine and may be a class effect. Additional studies are required to confirm these preliminary observations.

REFERENCES

Ahlfors UG, Baastrup PC, Dencker SJ, et al: Flupenthixol decanoate in recurrent manic depressive illness. A comparison with lithium. Acta Psychiatr Scand 64:226–237, 1981

Calabrese J, Keck PE Jr, Macfadden W, et al: A randomized, double-blind, placebo-controlled trial of quetiapine in the treatment of bipolar I or II depression. Am J Psychiatry 162:1351–1360, 2005

Gruber AJ, Cole JO: Antidepressant effects of flupenthixol. Pharmacotherapy 11:450–459, 1991

Keck PE Jr, McElroy SL, Strakowski SM, et al: Factors associated with maintenance antipsychotic treatment in patients with bipolar disorder. J Clin Psychiatry 57:147–151, 1996

Keck PE Jr, Marcus R, Tourkodimitris S, et al: A placebo-controlled, double-blind study of the efficacy and safety of aripiprazole in patients with acute bipolar mania. Am J Psychiatry 160:1651–1658, 2003a

Keck PE Jr, Versiani M, Potkin S, et al: Ziprasidone in the treatment of acute bipolar mania: a three-week, placebo-controled, double-blind, randomized trial. Am J Psychiatry 160:741–748, 2003b

Littlejohn R, Leslie F, Cookson J: Depot antipsychotics in the prophylaxis of bipolar affective disorder. Br J Psychiatry 165:827–829, 1994

Ozerdem A, Tunca Z, Kaya N: The relatively good prognosis of bipolar disorders in a Turkish bipolar clinic. J Affect Disord 64:27–34, 2001

Poldinger W, Sieberns S: Depression-inducing and antidepressive effects of neuroleptics. Experiences with flupenthixol and flupenthixol decanote. Neuropsychobiology 10:131–136, 1983

Sachs GS, Grossman F, Ghaemi SN, et al: Combination of a mood stabilizer with risperidone or haloperidol for treatment of acute mania: a double-blind, placebo-controlled comparison of efficacy and safety. Am J Psychiatry 159:1146–1154, 2002

Stark P, Hardison CD: A review of multicenter controlled studies of fluoxetine vs imipramine and placebo in outpatients with major depressive disorder. J Clin Psychiatry 46:53–58, 1985

Tohen M, Sanger TM, McElroy SL, et al: Olanzapine versus placebo in the treatment of acute mania. Am J Psychiatry 156:702–709, 1999

Tohen M, Jacobs TG, Grundy SL, et al: Efficacy of olanzapine in acute bipolar mania: a double-blind, placebo-controlled study. The Olanzapine HGGW Study Group. Arch Gen Psychiatry 57:841–849, 2000

Tohen M, Zhang F, Taylor CC, et al: A meta-analysis of the use of typical antipsychotic agents in bipolar disorder. J Affect Disord 65:85–93, 2001

Tohen M, Vieta E, Ketter T, et al: Efficacy of olanzapine and olanzapine-fluoxetine combination in the treatment of bipolar I depression. Arch Gen Psychiatry 60:1079–1088, 2003; erratum 61:176, 2004

Tohen M, Chengappa KN, Suppes T, et al: Relapse prevention in bipolar I disorder: 18-month comparison of olanzapine plus mood stabiliser v. mood stabiliser alone. Br J Psychiatry 184:337–345, 2004

Verdoux H, Gonzales B, Takei N, et al: A survey of prescribing practice of antipsychotic maintenance treatment for manic-depressive outpatients. J Affect Disord 38:81–87, 1996

Vieta E, Gastó C, Colom F, et al: Role of risperidone in bipolar II: an open 6-month study. J Affect Disord 67:213–219, 2001

White E, Cheung P, Silverstone T: Depot antipsychotics in bipolar affective disorder. Int Clin Psychopharmacol 8:119–122, 1993

Zarate CA Jr, Tohen M: Double-blind comparison of the continued use of antipsychotic treatment versus its discontinuation in remitted manic patients. Am J Psychiatry 161:169–171, 2004

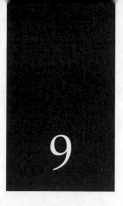

NOVEL TREATMENTS IN BIPOLAR DEPRESSION

Joseph Levine, M.D.

Julia Appelbaum, M.D.

Robert H. Belmaker, M.D.

TREATMENT FOR BIPOLAR DISORDER is currently characterized by polypharmacy, even in the best treatment centers (Kupfer et al. 2002)—many patients cannot be stabilized without it. In a prospective follow-up of a study by the Stanley Foundation Bipolar Network in which 258 bipolar patients were followed, Post et al. (2003) noted that two-thirds of these patients remained substantially affected by their illness despite treatment, with one-quarter remaining symptomatic for over 9 months. Patients were depressed three times as often as they were manic. These patients were being treated with polypharmacy as reflected by the use of an average of 4.4 psychotropic medications per patient (Post et al. 2003). The tendency for polypharmacy in the treatment of bipolar patients was also reported by Levine et al. (2000), who found that nearly 50% of bipolar patients received three or more psychotropic agents. Demographic characteristics appeared to have a minimal impact on prescription patterns.

Such a state of affairs calls for new approaches in the treatment of bipolar disorders. Given the time period these patients spend in the depressive phase, new modes and novel approaches to treatment are especially necessary. In this chapter, we present data on a variety of novel treatments for bipolar depression and review electroconvulsive therapy (ECT).

ATYPICAL NEUROLEPTICS

It has been suggested that typical antipsychotics increase the severity of depression or the number of depressive episodes in long-term maintenance treatment of bipolar patients (Keck et al. 1998; Kukopulos et al. 1980), although older literature from the 1950s and the 1960s suggested they may have antidepressive effects (Barsa and Kline 1957). Typical antipsychotics are also characterized by distressing side effects, including extrapyramidal side effects and tardive dyskinesia (Kane 1988).

A variety of atypical antipsychotics have repeatedly demonstrated beneficial effects in treatment-resistant depression, mainly as augmentation strategies (Barbee et al. 2004; Kennedy and Lam 2003; Masan 2004). Because treatments for unipolar depression are usually effective in bipolar depression, atypical antipsychotics are of increasing interest to those studying bipolar depression. Since the 1990s, preliminary data have suggested a role for atypical neuroleptics in the treatment of dysphoric mania or mixed mania: clozapine (McElroy et al. 1991), risperidone (Vieta et al. 1998), and olanzapine (Zullino and Baumann 1999) were reported in open studies to have some beneficial effects in dysphoric mania (see Chapter 8, "Antipsychotics in Bipolar Depression").

Clozapine

Clozapine was reported to have some effects on the dysphoric components of mania (Suppes et al. 1992). However, its antidepressant efficacy is not clear. The use of clozapine demands weekly monitoring, due to the 1%–2% incidence of agranulocytosis, and its use is reserved for patients with treatment-resistant conditions.

Risperidone

In open trials on patients with bipolar mania, risperidone therapy has led to significant reductions in depression scores compared with baseline. Four open-label studies of risperidone in bipolar subjects exhibiting mania, mixed state, or bipolar depression, were done in 2001–2003 (McIntyre and Katzman 2003; Vieta et al. 2001a, 2001b; Yatham et al. 2003). The Hamilton Rating Scale for Depression (Ham-D) or Montgomery-Åsberg Depression Rating Scale (MADRS) served as rating scales and risperidone was added to ongoing mood-stabilizing treatment. These studies examined the efficacy of risperidone for 3–6 months, demonstrating reduction of Ham-D or MADRS scores from baseline in patients with bipolar mania by 5–12 points.

Olanzapine

Vieta et al. (2001c) conducted an open study with olanzapine in a group of 23 bipolar type I and type II patients experiencing frequent relapses, residual subsyndromal symptoms, and inadequate responses to mood stabilizers, such as lithium, valproate, or carbamazepine. Treatment was maintained throughout the study. Last-observation-carried-forward analysis showed that after the introduction of olanzapine, there was a significant reduction of Clinical Global Impression (CGI) scores for both manic and depressive symptoms.

Reductions in depression scores in patients with bipolar mania have been significantly greater with olanzapine compared with placebo when olanzapine was administered as a monotherapy or as an add-on treatment to mood stabilizers (Tohen et al. 2002, 2003). Sanger et al. (2001) followed 113 bipolar patients previously participating in double-blind studies in a 49-week open-label extension phase. These patients demonstrated significant improvement in 21-item Ham-D scores along with antimanic effects. Baker et al. (2003) analyzed data from two similar placebo-controlled studies ($N=246$) of olanzapine in mania, focusing on depression scores in acutely ill manic patients with significant depressive symptoms ($n=86$). Olanzapine demonstrated a broad spectrum of efficacy, effectively treating both manic and depressive symptoms during mania. However, it is important to remember that depression during mania may be the same as isolated bipolar depression. It is important to specifically investigate the efficacy of treatment modalities in depressed, nonmanic, patients.

Olanzapine and Olanzapine-Fluoxetine Combination in the Treatment of Bipolar I Depression

Tohen et al. (2003) conducted a double-blind, 8-week, randomized, multisite, controlled trial of 833 adults with bipolar I depression with a MADRS score of at least 20 points. Patients were randomly assigned to receive placebo ($n=377$); 5–20 mg/day of olanzapine ($n=370$); or olanzapine-fluoxetine combination (OFC) 6 and 25 mg/day, 6 and 50 mg/day, or 12 and 50 mg/day ($n=86$). Olanzapine was found to be more effective than placebo but with a small, clinically insignificant effect size. OFC was found to be more effective than olanzapine and placebo in the treatment of bipolar I depression without increased risk of developing manic symptoms over the brief duration of the study. Shi et al. (2004) analyzed the above study for health-related, quality-of-life effects of these treatments and found that patients with bipolar depression receiving olanzapine or OFC for 8 weeks had greater improvement in health-related quality of life than those receiving placebo. OFC treatment was associated with greater improvement in health-related quality of life than olanzapine alone.

Comparing Risperidone and Olanzapine

McIntre et al. (2002) compared olanzapine with risperidone as an add-on to lithium or valproate for 6 months in 21 type I and II bipolar subjects in an open design. Ham-D scores served as a measure of depressive symptoms and significant reduction of Ham-D was noticed in both groups with no significant difference between them.

Quetiapine

Calabrese et al. (2005) reported on a study of 360 type I and 182 type II bipolar depressed patients receiving quetiapine monotherapy or placebo in a double-blind fashion for 8 weeks. Response rates for patients receiving 300 mg/day or 600 mg/day of quetiapine were 57.6% and 58.2%, respectively, significantly higher than 36.1% for placebo and only minimally smaller than the effect of antidepressants in unipolar depressive illness. Similarly, the remission rate (defined as MADRS<12) was significantly higher in the quetiapine-treated patients (52.9%) compared with placebo (28.4%). Separation from placebo was seen as early as the first week and remained significantly higher for the entire duration of the 8-week study (Calabrese et al. 2005).

An open-label, 12-week prospective study was conducted to assess the efficacy and tolerability of quetiapine in the treatment of patients with bipolar and schizoaffective disorder who were suboptimally responsive to mood stabilizers alone. The authors reported an overall improvement in these patients including a significant improvement in depressive symptoms (Sajatovic et al. 2001).

Altamura et al. (2003) reported on an open study of quetiapine in 28 bipolar patients. These patients received quetiapine or classical mood stabilizers at flexible doses for 12 months. Patients treated with both showed improvement of manic and depressive symptoms. Sokolski and Denson (2003) added quetiapine to bipolar patients who were partially responsive to lithium or valproate and found that quetiapine augmentation resulted in significant improvements in clinician-rated bipolar severity scores (CGI-BP) for both manic and depressive symptoms.

Ziprasidone

No controlled research data have been published on ziprasidone, an atypical drug also reported to inhibit reuptake of norepinephrine and serotonin (Schmidt et al. 2001). However, Papakostas et al. (2004) reported that ziprasidone can augment selective serotonin reuptake inhibitors (SSRIs) in SSRI-resistant major depressive disorder.

Summary

Preliminary studies suggest that atypical neuroleptics may exhibit some beneficial effects in bipolar depression. Most studies were uncontrolled or studied the effects of atypical neuroleptics on depressive symptoms in mixed bipolar patients. However, given the clear efficacy of typical antipsychotics in depression (whose clinical use was prevented mostly by extrapyramidal symptoms and tardive dyskinesia) it is likely that atypical antipsychotics will be increasingly useful in depression. If so, this may blur the traditional diagnostic boundaries between schizophrenia and affective disorder. It might also make the continuum between mania, mixed states, and depression less relevant to treatment.

ELECTROCONVULSIVE THERAPY

Electroconvulsive therapy (ECT) is an effective treatment for bipolar depression (Zornberg and Pope 1993). Several authors examined whether ECT is more effective in bipolar depression than in unipolar depression. Except for the results reported by Perris and d'Elia (1966), no advantage for bipolar depression over unipolar depression was found. Kukopulos et al. (1980) suggested that ECT, in contrast to tricyclic antidepressants, does not induce an accelerated course of bipolar illness. However, these authors reported that 39% of their patients developed mania while treated with ECT.

Srisurapanont et al. (1995) reviewed the literature on ECT treatment in bipolar depression. Although many studies did not differentiate between unipolar and bipolar depression, these authors concluded that ECT is considered by many to be a potent treatment for bipolar depression.

Ciapparelli et al. (2001) presented a study of ECT in medication-nonresponsive patients with mixed mania and bipolar depression. Forty-one patients with mixed mania and 23 patients with bipolar depression consecutively assigned to ECT treatment were included. Subjects were evaluated using the MADRS, the Brief Psychiatric Rating Scale (BPRS), and the Clinical Global Impressions-Severity of Illness (CGI-S) Scale. Assessments were carried out the day before starting ECT sessions, 48 hours after completion of the third session, and a week after the last session. Both groups received an equal number of ECT sessions. ECT treatment was associated with a substantial reduction in symptomatology, both in patients with mixed mania and in those with bipolar depression. However, the mixed mania group exhibited a more rapid and marked response as well as a greater reduction in suicidal ideation. Response to ECT was not influenced by the presence of delusions.

Grunhaus et al. (2002) reported the effectiveness of ECT in medication-nonresponsive patients with mixed mania and bipolar depression. There were 41 patients with mixed mania and 23 patients with bipolar depression. ECT was associated with a substantial reduction in symptomatology in both patient groups.

Interestingly, ECT may also induce mania. There is no clear answer in the literature whether mania induced by ECT can be further controlled if ECT is continued or its electrical parameters modified.

TRANSCRANIAL MAGNETIC STIMULATION

Transcranial magnetic stimulation (TMS) is being studied as a novel method of stimulating brain neurons in conscious humans (Hallett and Cohen 1989). Cortical magnetic stimulation can induce contralateral motor movements when applied to the motor strip (Hallett and Cohen 1989) and can induce speech arrest when administered over the speech area (Pascual-Leone et al. 1991). Magnetic stimulation has been used for many years for diagnostic purposes by neurologists.

The relatively recent development of stimulators capable of discharging at frequencies of up to 60 Hz has greatly expanded the applications for TMS in the cognitive and behavioral sciences. Depending on the stimulation frequency, intensity, and duration, trains of rapid-rate TMS (rTMS) can transiently block or inhibit the function of a given cortical region, and they can enhance the excitability of the affected cortical structures. It was proposed that stimulation over areas of the brain such as the prefrontal cortex might lead to emotional changes of possible therapeutic value in psychiatry (Belmaker and Fleischmann 1995). Uncontrolled (Grisaru et al. 1994) and controlled studies (George et al. 1996; Pascual-Leone et al. 1996) have reported antidepressant effects for TMS, especially left, prefrontal, rapid TMS. In normal controls, TMS has also been reported to cause mood changes specific to brain side in two separate controlled studies (Pascual-Leone et al. 1996). Paradoxically, studies of psychiatrically normal volunteers found increased sadness with left, prefrontal stimulation and increased happiness with right, prefrontal stimulation (Pascual-Leone et al. 1996).

Numerous studies have focused on evaluating efficacy and safety of TMS in unipolar depression, but only a small number of studies have been done in bipolar depression. Nahas et al. (2003) carried out a left prefrontal rTMS study focusing on determination of the safety, feasibility, and potential efficacy of using TMS to treat the depressive symptoms of bipolar affective disorder. Twenty-three patients were randomly assigned to receive either daily left prefrontal rTMS (5 Hz, 110% motor threshold, 8 seconds on, 22 seconds off, over 20 minutes) or placebo (sham rTMS) every morning for 2 weeks. No statistically significant difference between the two groups in the number of responders was found. Posttreatment, daily, subjective mood ratings showed a trend for improvement with active rTMS, compared with sham rTMS. In this pilot study, left prefrontal rTMS appeared safe in depressed bipolar subjects and the risk of inducing mania in such patients on medications was small.

Another controlled study of 20 patients with bipolar depression was carried out by Dolberg et al. (2002). Ten patients were treated with 20 sessions of left, prefrontal rTMS and the other ten received 10 sessions of sham TMS followed by 20 sessions of rTMS. Active rTMS was significantly superior to sham TMS with the most marked improvement after 2 weeks. No further improvement followed after 2 additional weeks of stimulation.

Tamas et al. (in press) performed a preliminary study of right-sided, slow rTMS. Slow (≤ 1 H$_3$) right rTMS may be effective in unipolar depression (Menkes et al. 1999). Only five patients were studied and, because of random assignment, only one patient received sham slow rTMS. There did not appear to be any difference at the end of 4 weeks (100 consecutive stimuli to right dorsolateral prefrontal cortex at 95% motor threshold, twice weekly). However, 2 weeks after treatment, there was an 11-point difference between active and placebo and a 13-point improvement in subjects receiving TMS.

A number of case reports of manic episodes following treatment with rTMS have been published (Dolberg et al. 2001; Garcia-Toro, 1999;

Sakkas et al. 2003). The total number of participants in these studies was small and additional research is necessary. Furthermore, the effect of right, prefrontal, slow TMS needs to be examined.

VAGUS NERVE STIMULATION

Vagus nerve stimulation (VNS) is an interesting procedure in which a pacemaker-like device is attached to an electrode that wraps around the left vagus in the lower neck (Rush et al. 2000). Periodic stimulation of the vagus alters functional activity in multiple regions of the brain (Chae et al. 2003).

Rush et al. (2005a) reported a randomized, sham-controlled study of VNS in treatment-resistant depression in 210 subjects with major depressive disorder and 25 bipolar depressed subjects. VNS and sham were administered for 10 weeks after a 2-week surgical recovery period. At the end of the study there was no significant difference in the primary outcome measure, the Ham-D. However, subjective improvement measured by the Inventory for Depressive Symptomatology–Self Report (IDS-SR$_{30}$) was significantly greater in the active group (17% response) versus the sham group (7.3% response, $P=0.03$) (Rush et al. 2005a). When these patients continued to receive active, open VNS in the ensuing 12 months ($n=185$ major depression, $n=20$ bipolar), 27.2% achieved remission (defined as a Ham-D score<9) (Rush et al. 2005b). There were an inadequate number of bipolar patients to perform a separate analysis. Three patients developed a mood shift. In two bipolar patients the episodes were mild: the patients were managed as outpatients, and the episodes resolved spontaneously. In the third patient, previously diagnosed with unipolar illness, the episode required hospitalization and lasted 2 months. All three patients had temporary discontinuation of the nerve stimulation which resumed after the episode (Rush et al. 2005b). Additionally, a case of hypomania following VNS for refractory epilepsy was previously reported (Klein et al. 2003). No other cases of mania or hypomania secondary to VNS have been reported.

George et al. (2005) openly compared treatment as usual (TAU; $n=124$) with VNS plus TAU ($n=205$) in treatment-resistant major depressive subjects (no bipolar subjects). At the end of 12 months, a significantly greater fraction of VNS plus TAU subjects (27%) achieved remission as defined by Ham-D reduction compared with those receiving TAU alone (13%, $P<0.01$).

Rush et al. (2000) examined the effects of VNS on treatment-resistant depressive patients. Adult outpatients ($N=30$) with nonpsychotic, treatment-resistant major depression ($n=21$) or bipolar depression type I ($n=4$) or type II ($n=5$) who had failed at least two medication trials in the current major depressive episode were treated with VNS for 10 weeks. Baseline 28-item Ham-D scores averaged 38 points. Response rates (>50% reduction in baseline scores) were 40% for the Ham-D and 50% for the MADRS. Symptomatic responses (accompanied by substantial functional improvement) have been largely sustained during long-term follow-up to date.

Sackeim et al. (2001) conducted an open pilot study of VNS in 60 patients with treatment-resistant major depressive episodes (MDEs) aimed to 1) define the response rate, 2) determine the profile of side effects, and 3) establish predictors of clinical outcome. Participants were outpatients with nonatypical, nonpsychotic, major depressive or bipolar disorder who had not responded to at least two medication trials from different antidepressant classes in the current MDE. VNS treatment lasted 10 weeks. Of 59 completers (one patient improved during the recovery period), the response rate was 30% for the primary 28-item Ham-D measure and 34% for the MADRS. The most common side effect was voice alteration or hoarseness (55%), which was generally mild and related to output current intensity. History of treatment resistance was predictive of VNS outcome. Patients who had never received ECT were four times more likely to respond. None of the 13 patients who had not responded to more than seven adequate antidepressant trials in the current MDE responded to VNS compared with 39% of the remaining 46 patients ($P=0.006$).

Therefore, VNS appears to be most effective in patients with low to moderate, but not extreme, antidepressant resistance. The authors state that evidence concerning long-term, therapeutic benefits and tolerability will be critical in determining the role of VNS in treatment-resistant depression (Rush et al. 2005a).

KETOGENIC DIET

The ketogenic diet (KD) has been used to treat epilepsy since the 1920s. The KD creates and maintains a state of ketosis as a result of changing the body's fuel from carbohydrates to fat. It is a treatment usually used in children with severe intractable epilepsy and has been found to be most effective for people with myoclonic seizures and minor motor seizures. It has also been helpful for people with tonic-clonic seizures and complex partial seizures. Although the diet seems to work best in children ages 1–10 years, it has also been used in adults (Levy and Cooper 2003; Thiele 2003).

There are two major types of this diet: the classic diet and the medium chain triglyceride (MCT) diet. The classic diet involves a ratio of 3:1 to 5:1 of fats to protein plus carbohydrates. The MCT diet patient usually obtains about 60% of their total calories from MCT oil. This diet, compared with the classic diet, allows more consumption of protein and carbohydrates.

Although the clinical efficacy of the KD in epilepsy is well documented, the underlying basis of KD antiepileptic efficacy is still unknown. Schwartzkroin (1999) summarized the theoretical background regarding the underlying mechanisms of KD suggesting five possible modes of action: 1) KD alters energy metabolism in the brain, thereby altering brain excitability; 2) KD leads to cellular changes that decrease excitability and dampen epileptiform discharge; 3) KD induces changes in neurotransmitter function and synaptic transmission, thereby altering inhibitory-excitatory balance and discouraging hyper-synchronization; 4) KD is associated with changes in a variety of circulating factors that act as neuromodulators that can regulate central nervous system excitability; and 5) KD gives rise to alterations in brain extracellular milieu, which serve to depress excitability and synchrony.

Ketogenic Diet and Bipolar Disorder

El-Mallakh and Paskitti (2001) suggested that the KD may be an effective mode of treatment for bipolar disorder. They hypothesized that the acidosis associated with the KD reduces intracellular sodium and intracellular free calcium, both of which are elevated in ill bipolar patients. However, Yaroslavsky et al. (2002) reported no beneficial effect of the KD in a case study of a bipolar woman. These authors applied a KD consisting of fats, carbohydrates, and protein in a 4:1 ratio (fats and carbohydrates to protein) to induce production of ketoacids in a slim, 49-year-old, physically healthy woman with severe, resistant, rapid-cycling bipolar disorder. The patient had early-onset bipolar disorder that deteriorated into continuous cycling episodes of manic-depressive illness without euthymic intervals. The patient was nonresponsive to lithium, carbamazapine, and valproic acid (individually or in combination) and the patient, her family, and the multidisciplinary staff agreed to KD treatment. Treatment with 10 mg/day of olanzapine was continued; she fasted for 48 hours and continued the classic KD for 2 weeks. No urinary ketosis or clinical improvement was noted and dietary fats were then replaced with MCT oil. Although the patient's compliance with the dietary restrictions was very good during the 1-month trial of KD, no clinical improvement was noticed, and there was no loss of weight and no urinary ketosis. The absence of urinary ketosis and the lack of ketone body measurements in blood raise questions as to whether an effective brain ketogenic metabolism was achieved in this patient. Further research is needed to sort out the feasibility and effectiveness of this treatment in various subgroups of bipolar patients.

Side Effects

Vitamin deficiency, hypocalcemia, and carnitine deficiency due to inadequate consumption of these agents have been reported in epilepsy studies (Levy and Cooper 2003). Other reported side effects include dehydration, constipation, and sometimes complications from kidney stones or gall stones (Levy and Cooper 2003). Adult women on the diet may have menstrual irregularities, pancreatitis, and decreased bone density (Levy and Cooper 2003). Excessive bruising and increase in minor bleeding in patients after institution of KD is probably associated with diet-induced changes in platelet function (Berry-Kravis et al. 2001). Recent studies have shown that the KD can also have some detrimental effects on cognitive ability (Zhao et al. 2004).

OMEGA-3 FATTY ACIDS

Omega-3 fatty acids are long-chain, polyunsaturated fatty acids (PUFA) found in plant and marine sources. PUFA seem also to exert intracellular effects on second messenger systems. Mirnikjoo et al. (2001) reported that omega-3 fatty acids could prevent serotonin receptor–induced mitogenic-activated protein kinase (MAPK) activation in hippocampal slice preparations. Results of studies from both in vitro and live cell preparations suggest that inhibition of second messenger–regulated protein kinases is one locus of action of omega-3 fatty acids.

In a cross-national comparison, Noaghiul and Hibbeln (2003) found a correlational relationship between greater seafood consumption and lower prevalence rates of bipolar disorders. However, research into the use of PUFAs in the treatment of bipolar disorder has lagged behind research regarding PUFAs as treatment for unipolar depression. To date, a number of open and controlled studies has been performed to examine whether omega-3 fatty acids are also useful in bipolar depression and exhibit mood-stabilizing properties in bipolar disorder. Chiu et al. (2003) have found significantly reduced arachidonic acid (20:4n-6) and docosahexaenoic acid (22:6n-3) compositions in bipolar patients as compared with normal controls. There were no differences in total omega-3 and omega-6 polyunsaturated fatty acids.

The first and best-known published study of omega-3 prophylaxis in bipolar disorders was reported by Stoll et al. (1999). These authors found that omega-3 fatty acids were well tolerated by patients, they improved the short-term course of illness, and resulted in a decreased incidence of depressive episodes. Su et al. (2003) reanalyzed the results reported in Stoll et al. (1999) and reported that most of the beneficial effects of omega-3 fatty acids were in the prevention of bipolar depression rather than mania.

In a study of patients with bipolar depression, Frangou and Lewis (2002) reported greater improvement in the omega-3 group compared with the placebo group (see Table 9–1). Keck and colleagues, in two separate clinical trials—one with bipolar hypomanic or depressed patients and another with bipolar depressed patients—found no benefit in adding eicosapentaenoic acid (EPA) daily to mood stabilizers (P.E. Keck Jr., M.P. Freeman, S. L. McElroy, et al., unpublished data, 2003) (see Table 9–1).

Osher et al. (2005) conducted an open-label add-on study of EPA (1.5–2 g/day) in outpatient bipolar patients with significant depressive symptomatology without psychotic features. Eight of the 10 patients who completed 1 month of EPA administration experienced a greater than 50% improvement on the Ham-D. However, the limitations of this study are its open-label design and a small sample size. It is encouraging that the bipolar clinical trials did not report omega-related switches to mania, although there is a case report in the literature which describes hypomania in a known bipolar patient, which may have been attributable to self-medication with omega-3 fatty acids (2 g/day of docosahexaenoic acid plus 1.3 g/day of EPA) (Kinrys 2000).

A number of issues connected to using PUFA in bipolar disorder remain unclear. Besides possible side effects, such as gastrointestinal effects and a fishy aftertaste, these fatty acids may induce prolonged bleeding time. Another unanswered curiosity is the relationship between the two active ingredients, EPA and docosahexaenoic acid (DHA): Why is it that smaller doses of EPA (1–2 g/day) seem to be more effective than larger doses, unless larger doses are combined with small doses of DHA? Also, it is not clear what is the optimal length of time required for good clinical response.

MYO-INOSITOL

Myo-inositol, a polyol, is an important brain osmolyte and a key precursor for the phosphatidylinositol (PI) second messenger cycle system

TABLE 9–1. Polyunsaturated fatty acids in bipolar depression

Study	Diagnosis	N	EPA g/day	DHA g/day	Results	Design
Keck et al. 2003	Bipolar depression	59	6	0	No benefit	Double blind, placebo controlled, add-on to mood stabilizer treatment
Keck et al. 2003	Bipolar (rapid cycling), hypomanic, or depression	62	6	0	No benefit	Double blind, placebo controlled, add-on treatment
Frangou et al. 2002	Bipolar depression	75	1 or 2	0	Greater improvement in omega group	Double-blind, placebo controlled, add-on treatment
Osher et al. 2005	Bipolar depression	12	2	0	2/3 of patients > 50% reduction on Ham-D within first month	Open, add-on treatment

Note. DHA = docosahexaenoic acid; EPA = eicosapentaenoic acid.

(Baraban et al. 1989). Levine et al. (1995) reported the administration of inositol to unipolar depressed patients in a double-blind, controlled trial. Inositol (12 g/day) or placebo was administered to 28 depressed patients for 4 weeks. The overall improvement in scores on the Ham-D was significantly greater for inositol than for placebo at week 4. No changes were noted in hematology or in kidney or liver function.

The PI cycle has been suggested as playing a pivotal role in bipolar disorders. Berridge et al. (1989) found that inositol depletion may be the key for lithium's effect in bipolar affective disorder. Williams et al. (2002) showed that all three mood stabilizers (lithium, valproic acid, and carbamazepine) inhibit the collapse of sensory neuron growth cones and increase growth cone area. These effects are reversible by inositol, thus implicating inositol depletion in the action of mood stabilizing agents. These data suggest that inositol depletion, like lithium, would be therapeutic in bipolar disorder. On the other hand, the encouraging results of inositol treatment in major depression suggest that inositol treatment might be therapeutic in bipolar depression.

Chengappa et al. (2000) studied 24 patients with bipolar depression ($n=21$, type I; $n=3$, type II) who were randomly assigned to receive either 12 g of inositol or D-glucose as placebo for 6 weeks. Efficacy and safety ratings were done weekly. Mood stabilizers (lithium, valproate, and carbamazepine) in stable doses and at therapeutic levels at study entry were continued unchanged. Twenty-two subjects completed the trial and 50% of the inositol-treated subjects ($n=12$) responded with a 50% or greater decrease in the baseline Ham-D score and a CGI scale score change of "much" or "very much" improved, as compared with 30% of the subjects administered placebo ($n=10$), a statistically nonsignificant difference. On the MADRS, 67% of inositol-treated subjects had a 50% or greater decrease in the baseline MADRS scores compared with 33% of subjects assigned to placebo ($P=0.10$). Inositol was well tolerated with minimal side effects, and thymoleptic blood levels were unaltered. These pilot data suggest that a controlled study with an adequate sample size may demonstrate efficacy for inositol in bipolar depression.

Evins et al. (2003) presented preliminary data of patients with bipolar type I or type II depression, despite receiving at least 2 weeks of therapeutic-level lithium or valproate, who were enrolled in a 6-week double-blind, placebo-controlled study of inositol versus placebo. The Ham-D and Young Mania Scale (YMS) were performed weekly. Sixteen subjects (baseline Ham-D score 24.6±3.6) were randomized; 9 received active inositol (mean dose 13.87±2.50 g/day) and 7 received placebo. Response criteria (> 50% reduction from baseline score in Ham-D at endpoint) were met by 33% of inositol-receiving subjects (95% CI=2.3%–63.7%)

and 0% of placebo-treated subjects (Fisher's exact test, $P=0.09$). YMS scores did not change significantly in either group. One placebo-treated subject was withdrawn from the study because of mania. No other serious adverse events occurred. Therefore, two different studies by two different groups support a small therapeutic effect of inositol in bipolar depression. Although both studies were of borderline statistical significance, they were both very small and underpowered to detect even a moderate effect size. The lack of pharmaceutical company support is probably the reason for the small size of these studies. Their consistent results and absence of side effects could encourage clinicians to try inositol in appropriate patients.

Interestingly, Antelman et al. (1998, 2000) reported that both inositol and lithium are effective in reducing the cyclicity in monoamine release induced by repeated cocaine administration in rat brain slices—a cycling model for bipolar illness.

DOPAMINE AGONISTS

From a phenomenological point of view, bipolar depression presents as an opposite to mania. Whereas bipolar depression shows retarded activity, slow thinking, and low mood, mania shows enhanced activity, rapid thinking, and heightened or irritable mood. Such dichotomous presentation of a disorder is rare in nature. Himmelhoch (2000) suggested that bipolar depression is centered around volitional inhibition and that there is a relationship between bipolar depression and involuntary motor disorders. Pharmacological agents effective in Parkinson's disease may be useful in bipolar depression. Such agents are mainly drugs affecting dopaminergic systems.

Pramipexole

Pramipexole, a dopamine agonist used to treat Parkinson's disease, was reported in two double-blind studies to be effective in bipolar depression (Goldberg et al. 2004; Zarate et al. 2004). Zarate et al. (2004) reported on the efficacy of pramipexole in bipolar type II depression. These authors conducted a double-blind, placebo-controlled study in 21 patients with DSM-IV-TR bipolar type II disorder, depressive phase. Patients were taking lithium or valproate at therapeutic levels and were randomly assigned to treatment with pramipexole ($n=10$) or placebo ($n=11$) for 6 weeks. All subjects, except for one in each group, completed the study. A therapeutic response (> 50% decrease in MADRS from baseline) occurred in 60% of patients taking pramipexole and 9% taking placebo, a statistically significant difference. One subject taking pramipexole and two receiving placebo developed hypomanic symptoms.

Goldberg et al. (2004) conducted a randomized, double-blind, placebo-controlled trial of pramipexole added to mood stabilizers for treatment-resistant bipolar depression. In this study, 22 depressed outpatients with DSM-IV-TR, nonpsychotic bipolar disorder were randomly assigned to receive placebo or a flexible dose of pramipexole added to existing mood stabilizers for 6 weeks. More patients given pramipexole (10 of 12) than patients given placebo (6 of 10) completed the study. Sixty-six percent patients taking pramipexole and only 20% taking placebo had an improvement of at least 50% in their Ham-D scores: the mean percentage of improvement from baseline was greater for patients taking pramipexole than for those taking placebo (48% vs. 21%). One patient developed hypomania while taking pramipexole.

These two studies suggest that pramipexole may have antidepressive effects in patients with bipolar depression. Larger randomized, controlled trials are needed to affirm these observations.

BRAIN ENERGY METABOLISM IN BIPOLAR DEPRESSION

Bipolar disorder as manifested by its opposite poles of depression and mania is characterized by decreased or increased motoric and mental energy expenditure. Does such a unique presentation suggest altered states of brain energy metabolism in this disorder?

Although the brain makes up about 2% of our total body weight, it consumes about 20% and 25% of total body dioxide and glucose, respectively. Neural activity is dependent upon energy metabolism mainly for the active transport of ions and other molecules through cellular membranes needed for neural excitation. Energy consumption is particularly high for Na^+/K^+-ATPase and Ca^{2+}-ATPase in plasma and endoplasmic membranes. Brain energy metabolism is reflected in adenosine-triphosphate (ATP) turnover. ATP, an energy-rich molecule with two high-energy phosphoanhydride bonds, is the energy donor in most energy-consuming processes, and its production in the brain is highly regulated. Another energy-rich molecule with high-energy phosphate is creatine phosphate, which enables the production of ATP from adenosine diphosphate via the creatine kinase/creatine phosphate system. This system may also function in regulating mitochondrial activity.

The key cellular organelle in cellular energy production is the mitochondrion. The electron flow in the mitochondria produces large amounts of energy converted into the chemical energy of ATP during oxidative phosphorylation in the mitochondria. The mechanisms of neuronal energy metabolism are not fully understood. Ames (2000) proposed the following percentages for energetic demands of neuronal key cellular processes: vegetative metabolism, 5%–15%; gated sodium influx through plasma membranes, 40%–50%; calcium influx from organelles, 3%–7%; processing of neurotransmitters, 10%–20%; intracellular signaling systems, 20%–30%; and axonal and dendritic transport 5%–15%. Agents decreasing the activity of gated sodium influx through plasma membranes or affecting second messenger intracellular systems may affect energy metabolism.

Positron emission tomography (PET) studies report reduced blood flow in depressed mood states, including bipolar depression (Baxter et al. 1985; Drevets et al. 1997; Ketter et al. 2001). PET studies reported lower fluorodeoxyglucose (FDG) uptake in the prefrontal and temporal cortexes and higher uptake in the occipital cortex of depressed patients compared with healthy controls, although in manic states the reverse direction of results was less clear. Single-photon emission computed tomography studies suggested lower cerebral blood flow in the frontal and temporal cortexes of bipolar disorder patients, particularly in the left hemisphere (Strakowski et al. 2000).

Magnetic resonance spectroscopy (MRS) provides a noninvasive window into brain neurochemistry. Decreased beta and total nucleotide triphosphate (primarily ATP) was reported in major depression in the frontal lobe (Volz et al. 1998) and basal ganglia (Moore et al. 1997). Kato et al. (1992) reported that creatine phosphate (CP)—but not ATP—is low in the frontal lobe of major depression patients; additionally, it was lower in severely depressed patients than in mildly depressed patients. These data suggest that depressive states may be associated with lower levels of high phosphorous energy metabolites.

Kato et al. (1994) reported reduction of brain phosphocreatine in bipolar disorder type II—but not in bipolar disorder type I—by the use of ^{31}P-MRS, which was found in the frontal lobes of patients during depressive, manic, and euthymic states. Kato et al. (1995) further noted a lateralized abnormality of high-energy phosphate metabolism in the frontal lobes of patients with bipolar disorder detected by phase-encoded ^{31}P-MRS reporting low CP levels in the left frontal lobe during depressive states. Yildiz et al. (2001) conducted a meta-analysis of ^{31}P-MRS studies in bipolar disorder supporting phospholipid and high-energy phosphate alterations in bipolar disorder that were primarily reflected by increased phosphomonoesters and decreased phospho-creatine in the depressed state, supporting abborent energy metabolism in bipolar illness.

Brain cellular pH was found to be decreased in bipolar disorder and it was suggested as being a state marker of altered brain energy metabolism, probably reflecting mitochondrial dysfunction. Increased lactate levels are generally associated with relatively low pH, and lactate is now also suggested as being involved in brain bioenergetics. Kato et al. (1998) reported decreased intracellular pH in euthymic patients, who are also drug free, whereas pH was normal in manic or depressive states. Hamakawa et al. (2004) reported reduced intracellular pH in the basal ganglia and whole brain measured by ^{31}P-MRS in bipolar disorder.

Dager et al. (2004) studied 32 medication-free patients with bipolar depression or with mixed mood state who showed elevated gray matter lactate and glutamine, glutamate, and γ-aminobutyric acid. An inverse correlation between the 17-item Ham-D and white matter creatine (creatine and phosphocreatine) was observed in bipolar patients. This implies a shift in energy metabolism from oxidative metabolism to glycolysis, possibly due to mitochondrial alterations.

Implications for Future Treatments

Future treatments of bipolar depression could be based on enhancing brain energy metabolism. Since oral creatine enters the brain and has been shown to raise brain creatine, we are conducting a study of creatine in bipolar depression.

REFERENCES

Altamura AC, Salvadori D, Madaro D, et al: Efficacy and tolerability of quetiapine in the treatment of bipolar disorder: preliminary evidence from a 12-month open-label study. J Affect Disord 76:267–271, 2003

Ames A 3rd: CNS energy metabolism as related to function. Brain Res Brain Res Rev 34:42–68, 2000

Antelman SM, Caggiula AR, Kucinski BJ, et al: The effects of lithium on a potential cycling model of bipolar disorder. Prog Neuropsychopharmacol Biol Psychiatry 22:495–510, 1998

Antelman SM, Levine J, Gershon S, et al: Is inositol likely to be effective in treating bipolar disorder? A prediction from a cycling model of the illness, in Basic Mechanisms and Therapeutic Implications of Bipolar Disorder. Edited by Soares JC, Gershon S. New York, Marcel Dekker, 2000, pp 49–58

Baker RW, Tohen M, Fawcett J, et al: Acute dysphoric mania: treatment response to olanzapine versus placebo. Clin Psychopharmacol 23:132–137, 2003

Baraban JM, Worley PF, Snyder SH: Second messenger systems and psychoactive drug action: focus on the phosphoinositide system and lithium. Am J Psychiatry 146:1251–1260, 1989

Barbee JG, Conrad EJ, Jamhour NJ: The effectiveness of olanzapine, risperidone, quetiapine, and ziprasidone as augmentation agents in treatment-resistant major depressive disorder. J Clin Psychiatry 65:975–981, 2004

Barsa JA, Kline NS: Depression treated with chlorpromazine and promethazine. Am J Psychiatry 113:744–745, 1957

Baxter LR Jr, Phelps ME, Mazziotta JC, et al: Cerebral metabolic rates for glucose in mood disorders. Studies with positron emission tomography and fluorodeoxyglucose F 18. Arch Gen Psychiatry 42:441–447, 1985

Belmaker RH, Fleischmann A: Transcranial magnetic stimulation: a potential new frontier in psychiatry. Biol Psychiatry 38:419–421, 1995

Berridge MJ, Downes CP, Hanley MR: Neural and developmental actions of lithium: a unifying hypothesis. Cell 59:411–419, 1989

Berry-Kravis E, Booth G, Taylor A, et al: Bruising and the ketogenic diet: evidence for diet-induced changes in platelet function. Ann Neurol 49:98–103, 2001

Calabrese JR, Keck PE Jr, Macfadden W, et al: A randomized, double-blind, placebo-controlled trial of quetiapine in the treatment of bipolar I or II depression. Am J Psychiatry 162:1351–1360, 2005

Chae JH, Nahas Z, Lomarev M, et al: A review of functional neuroimaging studies of vagus nerve stimulation (VNS). J Psychiatr Res 37:433–455, 2003

Chengappa KN, Levine J, Gershon S, et al: Inositol as an add-on treatment for bipolar depression. Bipolar Disord 2:47–55, 2000

Chiu CC, Huang SY, Su KP, et al: Polyunsaturated fatty acid deficit in patients with bipolar mania. Eur Neuropsychopharmacol 13:99–103, 2003

Ciapparelli A, Dell'Osso L, Tundo A, et al: Electroconvulsive therapy in medication-nonresponsive patients with mixed mania and bipolar depression. J Clin Psychiatry 62:552–555, 2001

Dager SR, Friedman SD, Parow A, et al: Brain metabolic alterations in medication-free patients with bipolar disorder. Arch Gen Psychiatry 61:450–458, 2004

Dolberg OT, Schreiber S, Grunhaus L: Transcranial magnetic stimulation-induced switch into mania: a report of two cases. Biol Psychiatry 49:468–470, 2001

Dolberg OT, Dannon PN, Schreiber S, et al: Transcranial magnetic stimulation in patients with bipolar depression: a double blind, controlled study. Bipolar Disord 4 (suppl 1):94–95, 2002

Drevets WC, Price JL, Simpson JR Jr, et al: Subgenual prefrontal cortex abnormalities in mood disorders. Nature 386:824–827, 1997

El-Mallakh RS, Paskitti ME: The ketogenic diet may have mood-stabilizing properties. Med Hypotheses 57:724–726, 2001

Evins EA, Nierenberg AA, Eisner L, et al: Inositol augmentation of mood stabilizers for bipolar depression. Paper presented at the Fifth International Conference for Bipolar Disorder, Pittsburgh, PA, June 12–14, 2003

Frangou S, Lewis M: The Maudsley bipolar disorder project: a double-blind, randomized, placebo-controlled study of ethyl-epa as an adjunct treatment of depression in bipolar disorder. Bipolar Disord 4:123, 2002

Garcia-Toro M: Acute manic symptomatology during repetitive transcranial magnetic stimulation in a patient with bipolar depression. Br J Psychiatry 175:491, 1999

George MS, Wassermann EM, Williams WA, et al: Changes in mood and hormone levels after rapid-rate transcranial magnetic stimulation (rTMS) of the prefrontal cortex. J Neuropsychiatry Clin Neurosci 8:172–180, 1996

George MS, Rush AJ, Marangell LB, et al: A one-year comparison of vagus nerve stimulation with treatment as usual for treatment-resistant depression. Biol Psychiatry 58:364–373, 2005

Goldberg JF, Burdick KE, Endick CJ: Preliminary randomized, double-blind, placebo-controlled trial of pramipexole added to mood stabilizers for treatment-resistant bipolar depression. Am J Psychiatry 161:564–566, 2004

Grisaru N, Yaroslavsky Y, Abarbanes J, et al: Transcranial magnetic stimulation in depression and schizophrenia. Eur Neuropsychopharmacol 4:287–288, 1994

Grunhaus L, Schreiber S, Dolberg OT, et al: Response to ECT in major depression: are there differences between unipolar and bipolar depression? Bipolar Disord 4 (suppl 1):91–93, 2002

Hallett M, Cohen LG: Magnetism: a new method for stimulation of nerve and brain. JAMA 262:538–541, 1989

Hamakawa H, Murashita J, Yamada N, et al: Reduced intracellular pH in the basal ganglia and whole brain measured by 31P-MRS in bipolar disorder. Psychiatry Clin Neurosci 58:82–88, 2004

Himmelhoch JM: Relationship of bipolar depression to involuntary motor disorders, in Basic Mechanisms and Therapeutic Implications. Edited by Soares JC, Gershon S. New York, Marcel Dekker, 2000, pp 317–342

Kane JM: The role of neuroleptics in manic-depressive illness. J Clin Psychiatry 49(suppl):12–14, 1988

Kato T, Takahashi S, Shioiri T, et al: Brain phosphate metabolism in patients with manic-depressive psychosis [in Japanese]. Seishin Shinkeigaku Zasshi 94:972–976, 1992

Kato T, Takahashi S, Shioiri T, et al: Reduction of brain phosphocreatine in bipolar II disorder detected by phosphorus-31 magnetic resonance spectroscopy. J Affect Disord 31:125–133, 1994

Kato T, Shioiri, T, Murashita J: Lateralized abnormality of high energy phosphate metabolism in the frontal lobes of patients with bipolar disorder detected by phase-encoded ^{31}P-MRS. Psychol Med 25:557–566, 1995

Kato T, Murashita J, Kamiya A, et al: Decreased brain intracellular pH measured by ^{31}P-MRS in bipolar disorder: a confirmation in drug-free patients and correlation with white matter hyperintensity. Eur Arch Psychiatry Clin Neurosci 248:301–306, 1998

Keck PE Jr, McElroy SL, Strakowski SM: Anticonvulsants and antipsychotics in the treatment of bipolar disorder. J Clin Psychiatry 59 (suppl 6):74–81, (discussion 82), 1998

Kennedy SH, Lam RW: Enhancing outcomes in the management of treatment resistant depression: a focus on atypical antipsychotics. Bipolar Disord 5 (suppl 2):36–47, 2003

Ketter TA, Kimbrell TA, George MS, et al: Effects of mood and subtype on cerebral glucose metabolism in treatment-resistant bipolar disorder. Biol Psychiatry 49:97–109, 2001

Kinrys G: Hypomania associated with omega3 fatty acids. Arch Gen Psychiatry 57:715–716, 2000

Klein JP, Jean-Baptiste M, Thompson JL, et al: A case report of hypomania following vagus nerve stimulation for refractory epilepsy. J Clin Psychiatry 64:485, 2003

Kukopulos A, Reginaldi D, Laddomada P, et al: Course of the manic-depressive cycle and changes caused by treatment. Pharmakopsychiatr Neuropsychopharmakol 13:156–167, 1980

Kupfer DJ, Frank E, Grochocinski VJ, et al: Demographic and clinical characteristics of individuals in a bipolar disorder case registry. J Clin Psychiatry 63:120–125, 2002; comment 63:1045–1046; author reply 63:1046, 2002

Levine J, Barak Y, Gonzalves M, et al: Double-blind, controlled trial of inositol treatment of depression. Am J Psychiatry 152:792–794, 1995

Levine J, Chengappa KN, Brar JS, et al: Psychotropic drug prescription patterns among patients with bipolar I disorder. Bipolar Disord 2:120–130, 2000

Levy R, Cooper P: Ketogenic diet for epilepsy. Cochrane Database Syst Rev CD001903, 2003

Masan PS: Atypical antipsychotics in the treatment of affective symptoms: a review. Ann Clin Psychiatry 16:3–13, 2004

McElroy SL, Dessain EC, Pope HG Jr, et al: Clozapine in the treatment of psychotic mood disorders, schizoaffective disorder, and schizophrenia. J Clin Psychiatry 52:411–414, 1991

McIntre R, Mancini DA, McCann SM, et al: Antidepressant efficacy and tolerability of risperidone and olanzapine in bipolar disorder. Presented at the XXIII Congress of the Collegium Internationale Neuro-Psychopharmalogicium, Montreal, Canada, MONTH 2002

McIntyre R, Katzman M: The role of atypical antipsychotics in bipolar depression and anxiety disorders. Bipolar Disord 5 (suppl 2):20–35, 2003

Mirnikjoo B, Brown SE, Kim HF, et al: Protein kinase inhibition by omega-3 fatty acids. J Biol Chem 276:10888–10896, 2001

Moore CM, Christensen JD, Lafer B, et al: Lower levels of nucleoside triphosphate in the basal ganglia of depressed subjects: a phosphorous-31 magnetic resonance spectroscopy study. Am J Psychiatry 154:116–118, 1997

Nahas Z, Kozel FA, Li X, et al: Left prefrontal transcranial magnetic stimulation (TMS) treatment of depression in bipolar affective disorder: a pilot study of acute safety and efficacy. Bipolar Disord 5:40–47, 2003

Noaghiul S, Hibbeln JR: Cross-national comparisons of seafood consumption and rates of bipolar disorders. Am J Psychiatry 160:2222–2227, 2003

Osher Y, Bersudsky Y, Belmaker RH: Omega-3 eicosapentaenoic acid in bipolar depression: report of a small open-label study. J Clin Psychiatry 66:726–729, 2005

Papakostas GI, Petersen TJ, Nierenberg AA, et al: Ziprasidone augmentation of selective serotonin reuptake inhibitors (SSRIs) for SSRI-resistant major depressive disorder. J Clin Psychiatry 65:217–221, 2004

Pascual-Leone A, Gates JR, Dhuna A: Induction of speech arrest and counting errors with rapid-rate transcranial magnetic stimulation. Neurology 41:697–702, 1991

Pascual-Leone A, Rubio B, Pallardo F, et al: Rapid-rate transcranial magnetic stimulation of left dorsolateral prefrontal cortex in drug-resistant depression. Lancet 348:233–237, 1996

Perris C, d'Elia G: A study of bipolar (manic-depressive) and unipolar recurrent depressive psychoses. IX: therapy and prognosis. Acta Psychiatr Scand Suppl 194:153–171, 1966

Post RM, Denicoff KD, Leverich GS, et al: Morbidity in 258 bipolar outpatients followed for 1 year with daily prospective ratings on the NIMH life chart method. J Clin Psychiatry 64:680–690, 2003

Rush AJ, George MS, Sackeim HA, et al: Vagus nerve stimulation (VNS) for treatment-resistant depressions: a multicenter study. Biol Psychiatry 47:276–286, 2000

Rush AJ, Marangell LB, Sackeim HA, et al: Vagus nerve stimulation for treatment-resistant depression: a randomized, controlled acute phase trial. Biol Psychiatry 58:347–354, 2005a

Rush AJ, Sackeim HA, Sackeim HA, et al: Effects of 12 months of vagus nerve stimulation in treatment-resistant depression: a naturalistic study. Biol Psychiatry 58:355–363, 2005b

Sackeim HA, Rush AJ, George MS, et al: Vagus nerve stimulation (VNS) for treatment-resistant depression: efficacy, side effects, and predictors of outcome. Neuropsychopharmacology 25:713–728, 2001

Sajatovic M, Brescan DW, Perez DE, et al: Quetiapine alone and added to a mood stabilizer for serious mood disorders. J Clin Psychiatry 62:728–732, 2001

Sakkas P, Mihalopoulou P, Mourtzouhou P, et al: Induction of mania by rTMS: report of two cases. Eur Psychiatry 18:196–198, 2003

Sanger TM, Grundy SL, Gibson PJ, et al: Long-term olanzapine therapy in the treatment of bipolar I disorder: an open-label continuation phase study. J Clin Psychiatry 62:273–281, 2001

Schmidt AW, Lebel LA, Howard HR Jr, et al: Ziprasidone: a novel antipsychotic agent with a unique human receptor binding profile. Eur J Pharmacol 425:197–201, 2001

Schwartzkroin PA: Mechanisms underlying the anti-epileptic efficacy of the ketogenic diet. Epilepsy Res 37:171–180, 1999

Shi L, Namjoshi MA, Swindle R, et al: Effects of olanzapine alone and olanzapine/fluoxetine combination on health-related quality of life in patients with bipolar depression: secondary analyses of a double-blind, placebo-controlled, randomized clinical trial. Clin Ther 26:125–134, 2004

Sokolski KN, Denson TF: Adjunctive quetiapine in bipolar patients partially responsive to lithium or valproate. Prog Neuropsychopharmacol Biol Psychiatry 27:863–866, 2003

Srisurapanont M, Yatham LN, Zis AP: Treatment of acute bipolar depression: a review of the literature. Can J Psychiatry 40:533–544, 1995

Stoll AL, Severus WE, Freeman MP: Omega 3 fatty acids in bipolar disorder: a preliminary double-blind, placebo-controlled trial. Arch Gen Psychiatry 56:407–412, 1999

Strakowski SM, DelBello MP, Adler C, et al: Neuroimaging in bipolar disorder. Bipolar Disord 2:148–164, 2000

Su KP, Huang SY, Chiu CC, et al: Omega-3 fatty acids in major depressive disorder: a preliminary double-blind, placebo-controlled trial. Eur Neuropsychopharmacol 13(4):267–271, 2003

Suppes T, McElroy SL, Gilbert J, et al: Clozapine in the treatment of dysphoric mania. Biol Psychiatry 32:270–280, 1992

Tamas RL, Menkes D, El-Mallakh RS: Stimulating research: a prospective, randomized, double-blind, sham controlled study of slow transcranial magnetic stimulation in depressed bipolar patients. J Neuropsychiatry Clin Neurosci (in press)

Thiele EA: Assessing the efficacy of antiepileptic treatments: the ketogenic diet. Epilepsia 44 (suppl 7):26–29, 2003

Tohen M, Chengappa KN, Suppes T, et al: Efficacy of olanzapine in combination with valproate or lithium in the treatment of mania in patients partially nonresponsive to valproate or lithium monotherapy. Arch Gen Psychiatry 59:62–69, 2002

Tohen M, Vieta E, Calabrese J, et al: Efficacy of olanzapine and olanzapine-fluoxetine combination in the treatment of bipolar I depression. Arch Gen Psychiatry 60:1079–1088, 2003

Vieta E, Gasto C, Colom F, et al: Treatment of refractory rapid cycling bipolar disorder with risperidone. J Clin Psychopharmacol 18(2):172–174, 1998

Vieta E, Gasto C, Colom F, et al: Role of risperidone in bipolar II: an open 6-month study. J Affect Disord 67:213–219, 2001a

Vieta E, Goikolea JM, Corbella B, et al: Risperidone safety and efficacy in the treatment of bipolar and schizoaffective disorders: results from a 6-month, multicenter, open study. J Clin Psychiatry 62:818–825, 2001b

Vieta E, Reinares M, Corbella B, et al: Olanzapine as long-term adjunctive therapy in treatment-resistant bipolar disorder. J Clin Psychopharmacol 21:469–473, 2001c

Volz HP, Rzanny R, Riehemann S, et al: ^{31}P magnetic resonance spectroscopy in the frontal lobe of major depressed patients. Eur Arch Psychiatry Clin Neurosci 248:289–295, 1998

Williams RS, Cheng L, Mudge AW, et al: A common mechanism of action for three mood-stabilizing drugs. Nature 417:292–295, 2002

Yaroslavsky Y, Stahl Z, Belmaker RH: Ketogenic diet in bipolar illness. Bipolar Disord 4:75, 2002

Yatham LN, Binder C, Riccardelli R, et al: Risperidone in acute and continuation treatment of mania. Int Clin Psychopharmacol 18:227–235, 2003

Yildiz A, Sachs GS, Dorer DJ, et al: ^{31}P Nuclear magnetic resonance spectroscopy findings in bipolar illness: a meta-analysis. Psychiatry Res 106:181–191, 2001

Zarate CA, Jr, Payne JL, Singh J, et al: Pramipexole for bipolar II depression: a placebo-controlled proof of concept study. Biol Psychiatry 56:54–60, 2004

Zhao Q, Stafstrom CE, Fu DD, et al: Detrimental effects of the ketogenic diet on cognitive function in rats. Pediatr Res 55:498–506, 2004

Zornberg GL, Pope HG Jr: Treatment of depression in bipolar disorder: new directions for research. J Clin Psychopharmacol 13:397–408, 1993

Zullino D, Baumann P: Olanzapine for mixed episodes of bipolar disorder. J Psychopharmacol 13:198, 1999

PSYCHOLOGICAL INTERVENTIONS IN BIPOLAR DEPRESSION

Francesc Colom, Psy.D., M.Sc., Ph.D.
Eduard Vieta, M.D., Ph.D.

THE LAST 5 YEARS HAVE BEEN crucial for the study of psychological treatment as a powerful add-on to medication in the prophylactic treatment of bipolar disorders. After many years of speculation and little evidence, several studies published in outstanding scientific journals showed the efficacy of several psychological approaches in preventing relapses into mania or depression. Training in prodromal identification (Perry et al. 1999), family-focused interventions (Miklowitz et al. 2003), cognitive-behavioral therapy (Lam et al. 2003), and psychoeducation (Colom et al. 2003a, 2003b) reached more than acceptable results in randomized clinical trials. Today, treatment guidelines include psychological interventions as a regular tool for maintaining euthymia (Calabrese et al. 2004; Goodwin et al. 2003). However, when looking at the efficacy of psychotherapy in the acute phases of bipolar illness, we may find a very different scenario (i.e., psychotherapy actually has acute efficacy in bipolar depression). Although several psychological interventions have shown efficacy in preventing mania (Colom et al. 2003a; Lam et al. 2003; Perry et al. 1999), any sort of psychological therapy for acutely manic patients appears to be an unlikely treatment option given the striking efficacy of newer antimanic agents, which leaves little room for non-pharmacological approaches other than electroconvulsive therapy (ECT) for treatment-resistant mania. This is not the case for bipolar depression, for which there are a number of reasons that tailored psychological strategies with demonstrated efficacy are needed to complement pharmacotherapy (see Table 10–1).

Interestingly, the combination of psychotherapy and antidepressants was mentioned as the first choice in the treatment of bipolar depression in a survey performed with Canadian psychiatrists (Sharma et al. 1997). According to this study, only 15% of psychiatrists would start treating bipolar depression with medication alone. Some 20% of psychiatrists would choose a cognitive-behavioral intervention, and just 5% mentioned psychoeducation as a choice. Unfortunately, in the same survey, half of the participants would choose what they called "eclectic" psychotherapy, although they did not properly define the term (making any interpretation of efficacy nearly meaningless), and we currently have no studies based on this so-called approach. Readers should keep in mind that this study was performed before 1999, when bipolar psychotherapy started to become accepted and widely practiced; if this survey were repeated today, the results might indicate the use of evidence-based approaches such as cognitive-behavioral interventions or interpersonal therapy. Regardless, the message for clinical psychologists and psychotherapy experts is quite clear: psychiatrists are not using any sort of criteria in choosing a certain type of psychotherapy for treatment of bipolar depression; instead, they are depending only on intuition. This reliance on intuition alone can readily be ascribed to the lack of randomized clinical trials in the field of clinical psychology throughout the last few decades. In other words, psychiatrists do not regularly use evidence-based criteria when deciding to include particular psychological treatments for certain symptomatologies because there are not enough data from well-designed studies on which to base such criteria. While pharmacotherapy research has made a strong effort in showing its efficacy through well-designed studies, psychotherapy research has focused more on persuading clinicians through arguments beyond science. It has been shown that once psychologists have demonstrated the prophylactic efficacy of their interventions in bipolar disorders (e.g., Colom et al. 2003a; Lam et al. 2003; Miklowitz et al. 2003), there is little reluctance by psychiatrists to include them as a treatment choice—even in their psychopharmacological guidelines (Goodwin et al. 2003).

Although the evidence is still scanty, there are currently two promising approaches in the treatment of bipolar depression: cognitive-behavioral

---

TABLE 10–1. Reasons for considering psychological interventions in bipolar depression

---

- Depression and depressive cycling remain a substantial problem in about two-thirds of intensively treated bipolar outpatients (Post et al. 2003).
- Bipolar depression is the predominant abnormal affective pole and causes greater disability and economic burden than mania (Bowden and Krishnan 2004).
- Symptoms of bipolar depression occur more frequently, last longer, are more disruptive, and are associated with greater risk of suicide than symptoms of mania (Hirschfeld 2004).
- Some studies suggest an unfavorable cost/benefit ratio for antidepressant treatment of bipolar depression (Ghaemi et al. 2004).
- Antidepressants have not been shown to definitively prevent completed suicides and reduce mortality (Ghaemi et al. 2003).
- Antidepressants carry the risk of inducing a switch and should be reserved for severe cases; they should not be routinely used in mild to moderate cases (Ghaemi et al. 2003). However, see Vieta 2003 for an opposing view.
- Bipolar patients have significantly lower self-esteem compared with controls (Blairy et al. 2004), which can be improved by several types of psychotherapy.

---

therapy (CBT) and interpersonal social rhythm therapy (IPSRT). Both treatments have proven efficacy in unipolar depression, and most clinicians accept them as useful strategies when treating a nonpsychotic bipolar depression, despite the fact that we still need definite, randomized, controlled studies to ascertain their real efficacy (Frances et al. 1998).

U.S. treatment guidelines consider psychological interventions as a second choice in the treatment of bipolar depression, immediately after the optimization of mood stabilizers and at the same level as antidepressants or ECT (American Psychiatric Association 2002). From a European perspective, we may be not so optimistic regarding this privileged position; psychotherapy is, undoubtedly, a very safe treatment in terms of avoiding switch-risk, but little is known about its outcome. Therefore, we should need to carefully consider the relationship between safety and efficacy in depressive patients, especially given the high suicide rates associated with bipolar depression, which would justify a more ambitious intervention (Vieta 2003). With this is mind, we would never consider psychotherapy as being at the same level as antidepressants or ECT, mainly because the responder's clinical profile is different for each treatment. For instance, we would consider psychotherapy as an add-on first-line treatment in the case of mild or moderate depression in rapid-cycling patients or patients with bipolar disorder type III (i.e., patients with antidepressant-induced mania), in whose treatment caution in the use of antidepressants is especially recommended because of the risk of inducing a switch. However, there is little data to back this assertion, and the availability of lamotrigine may change the panorama a bit. We do not exclude treatment algorithms of psychological interventions for treating severe bipolar depression; together with antidepressants and mood stabilizers, psychotherapy may play a very important role in preventing suicide and helping patients cope with dysfunctional attitudes and behaviors.

The U.S. guidelines mentioned above reflect what is a common opinion among many clinicians—namely, that psychotherapy would be especially useful for those patients with psychosocial triggering factors. In our opinion, reducing the indication of psychological interventions exclusively to episodes triggered by adverse events is highly unspecific, too restrictive, and would limit the indication of psychological interventions to first depressive episodes because subsequent episodes could be interpreted as being spontaneous or induced by medication. Furthermore, although there are no data available on the efficacy of psychotherapy in treating dysphoria or hypothymia that usually follows mania, some authors consider cognitive therapy as the first treatment choice for such symptoms (Jacobs 1982).

COGNITIVE-BEHAVIORAL THERAPY IN BIPOLAR DEPRESSION

The efficacy of CBT in the treatment of unipolar depression is unquestionable, both in combination therapy and in monotherapy (Keller et al. 2000; Scott et al. 2000; Ward et al. 2000). However, these results should not be generalized to bipolar depression because the two have subtle but relevant clinical differences. Bipolar depression is often characterized by hypersomnia, inhibition, lethargy, and apathy (mainly behavioral symptoms) whereas unipolar depression is defined by desperation, pessimistic thoughts, and other cognitive signs (Goodwin and Jamison 1990). Although it is true that cognitive symptoms are not absent in bipolar depression, they may be more typical of unipolar depression. Therefore, bipolar depression would better respond to a behavioral therapy focused on activation, whereas a classical, cognitive therapy would be more appropriate for unipolar patients. (For this reason, we will refer to CBT as *BCT* from this point on because we believe that the behavioral strategies are much more important than the cognitive strategies in the treatment of bipolar disorder and therefore should be the first indicated in the name of the treatment.)

This difference has been largely overlooked by experts coming from orthodox, academic cognitive schools, who have unsuccessfully tried to treat bipolar depression following the classic Beck's model (Leahy and Beck 1988). In the field of psychotherapy, an academic position on a particular treatment regarding severe mental disorders usually encounters problems finding supportive clinical evidence, primarily because mastering a model does not necessarily mean understanding a certain illness. Basically, cognitive-behavioral therapy assumes that maladaptive behavior and certain cognitive patterns cause psychiatric symptoms. The treatment focuses on changing these patterns through a logical discussion or behavioral activation in order to improve symptoms. The problem with adapting this assumption of cognitive patterns as a cause of symptoms to bipolar disorder is that it is, simply, not true: cognitive patterns are not *causing* emotions in bipolar depression. In most bipolar patients there is no cognitive change; if there is one, it is best described as being modified by the emotional state: cognitive changes are more likely the consequence than the cause of bipolar depression.

It would be very interesting to compare the efficacy of "pure" cognitive therapy versus behavioral therapy in the field of bipolar depression—although from a "behavioral" position this study would be almost impossible, because cognition is behavior. Currently, the number of studies on bipolar BCT is so small that we could not say exactly what future studies would be most relevant and helpful in supplementing the current body of work.

There is some ambiguity with respect to the meaning of terms for psychological interventions. *Psychoanalysis* includes a wide variety of very different interventions, as does *cognitive-behavioral*. Although classic BCT has never shown any evidence in the treatment of bipolar depression, there are some promising studies on the efficacy of some cognitive/psychoeducational strategies—labeled BCT as well—both as a treatment for acute bipolar depression and as a prophylactic add-on (Lam et al. 2003). The most remarkable study on BCT as a treatment of bipolar depression is reported in Scott et al. (2001). In this study, 42 patients were randomized to receive either immediate cognitive therapy or 6 months on a waiting list to be followed by cognitive therapy. After 6 months, those who had already received cognitive therapy had significantly greater improvements in depressive symptoms, as measured by the Beck Depression Inventory (BDI). Six months after cognitive therapy had ended, there was only a slight but nonsignificant increase in symptoms from the point at which therapy had ended. The authors emphasized that cognitive intervention was more complex for bipolar than for unipolar patients, but the results they obtained are especially encouraging given the difficulty of treating bipolar depression with medication alone, the switch risk, and the suicide rates. The same study also suggests the efficacy of BCT in improving subthreshold symptoms.

Several preliminary studies show the feasibility of BCT as treatment for bipolar depression and suggest its implementation in treatment routines, though these reports are generally based on a small sample size (Palmer and Williams 1995; Patelis-Siotis et al. 2001). The same pitfall seriously hinders the conclusions from other studies trying to assess the efficacy of BCT in improving bipolar depressive symptoms (Zaretsky et al. 1999).

BCT also may be efficacious for treating postmanic periods (Jacobs 1982). After a hypomanic or manic phase, the patient may look hypoactive and abulic. In these cases antidepressant treatment should be avoided because there may be a risk of inducing a switch into mania or rapid cycling (Wehr 1993). Self-control techniques, stress management and inoculation, exposition, and coping might be useful in the treatment of specific problems derived from illness.

A common element of every psychotherapy that works in treating bipolar disorders is that the rationale is completely based on clinical experience and common sense. Although showing the most obvious evidence will always be a part of scientific studies and, consequently, randomized, clinical trials will always be indispensable, the truth is that good clinicians can know what is likely good practice through experience—for example, many clinicians knew that informing the family is good for the patient long before David Miklowitz reported evidence for this assertion (Miklowitz et al. 2003), and the same can be said about psychoeducation or cognitive approaches. Behavioral modification of patient routines is probably the most frequently used pragmatic approach in clinical practice, with no thought given to formally assessing its efficacy. Therefore, with a depressed bipolar patient, one does not need to be a BCT expert to encourage activation, advise a reduction of sleeping time, or promote exercise—it is simply common sense. Unfortunately, just a few papers concern the usefulness of common sense in psychotherapy.

Among the behavioral interventions that have traditionally been used to approach depression, sleep deprivation showed strong efficacy rates—40%–75% of patients improved (Schilgen and Tolle 1980), but most of the patients (50%–80%) relapsed after sleep regulation (Giedke and Schwarzler 2002). To the best of our knowledge, the only existing study on sleep deprivation including bipolar spectrum patients is the

Heim study (1988), which compared 50 bipolar and cyclothymic patients receiving bright-light treatment with 50 bipolar and cyclothymic patients receiving partial sleep deprivation; the results were slightly superior for the bright-light treatment group. Unfortunately, the study does not include a placebo arm, and it is impossible to obtain any therapeutic outcome from such methodology. Sleep-deprivation may not be an appropriate intervention for bipolar depression but behavioral strategies for reducing the number of sleeping hours are largely advised.

INTERPERSONAL SOCIAL RHYTHM THERAPY

Interpersonal social rhythm therapy illustrates another problem in terminology. Interpersonal therapy was formerly known as a psychodynamic approach developed by Harry Stack Sullivan. Psychodynamic interpersonal therapy inspired Gerald Klerman and his team (1984), who reformulated a newer "behaviorally focused" interpersonal therapy that allowed a simple and reliable assessment of its results and was time limited. These characteristics enabled IPSRT—an adaptation of the Klerman interpersonal therapy developed by the Pittsburgh group (Frank et al. 1990) to address the needs of bipolar patients—to become a desirable standard for psychological interventions in bipolar disorders. The efficacy of IPSRT on unipolar depression has been widely proven (Elkin et al. 1989, 1995; Frank et al. 1991), and data on bipolar depression are quite promising: patients receiving IPSRT experienced less depressive relapses, earlier recovery from depression, and less subthreshold depressive symptomatology than patients assigned to other treatment conditions (Frank 1999; Frank et al. 1999; Miklowitz et al. 2000). IPSRT has been shown to be efficacious for reducing the risk of bipolar suicide (Rucci et al. 2002), but further studies are urgently needed to ascertain its efficacy in the treatment of bipolar depression.

PSYCHOTHERAPY TREATMENT OF NUCLEAR SYMPTOMS AND ASSOCIATED PROBLEMS

One of the main prejudices that many psychiatrists have toward clinical psychology is that psychotherapy does not work with core symptoms and that it is useful only for associated problems or for understanding triggering factors, thereby limiting the role of psychological intervention to one of simply supporting the patient. Nevertheless, psychological interventions have shown efficacy in improving some serious nuclear conditions, such as the number of relapses (Colom et al. 2003a; Lam et al. 2003), providing hope that this might also be the case for bipolar depression.

Associated Problems

There are several problems often associated with bipolar disorders that may worsen the quality of life of patients and therefore deserve special attention. Patients may run into problems during their adjustment to a diagnosis; common reactions to receiving a diagnosis of a severe, chronic illness are denial, anger, ambivalence, and anxiety (Goodwin and Jamison 1990). It is essential for the clinician to respond appropriately in order to to improve illness awareness, treatment compliance, and avoid self-esteem problems (Colom and Vieta 2002a, 2002b). Another problem that should be carefully addressed by therapists is a patient's feeling of loss and grief after the loss of real or abstract objects, such as a job (which is mentioned by 70% of patients and their partners as the most relevant difficulty in the long term [Targum et al. 1981]), job status (which affects more than 30% of patients [Harrow et al. 1990]), economic status, and loss of love relationships and family support. All of these losses are often followed by intense feelings of guilt, derived from a subtle form of poor illness insight, in which the patient has a false expectation of control over his or her symptoms that becomes frustration when the patient realizes that it is completely impossible to maintain a stable mood without medication. All of these losses are reactivated during the depressive phase and should be approached during a psychotherapy, including psychoeducation. The loss of abstract objects includes grief for the loss of the healthy self, most frequently occurring in anxious patients overinvolved in their own illness. Regular psychoeducation is not the first choice of treatment for this type of patient; a cognitive approach is recommended when overinvolvement appears. Grief for the healthy self may be observed as a dysfunctional assumption worsening the course of bipolar disorder, as recently reported by Lam et al. (2004).

Depressive Core Symptoms

Any psychological treatment approaching bipolar depression should include behavioral activation and daily restructuring activities to cope with apathy and lack of energy—two common symptoms of bipolar depression. Therefore, behavioral therapy is often indicated, although IPSRT would be another possible choice. For patients with nonmelancholic bipolar depression it is especially useful to begin psychotherapy. Previously psychoeducated depressed patients usually respond promptly to the behavioral instructions of their therapists because they have already assumed a medical model of their illness and cognitions are usually less altered.

Regarding anxiety management, common in bipolar depression and in many other phases of the illness, it is worth mentioning that, to some extent, most psychotherapeutic programs include behavioral techniques such as muscle relaxation. However, anxiety during bipolar depression mostly has to do with feelings of guilt associated to apathy. Thus, a cognitive approach would be very useful to cope with this feature.

Studies on the behavioral-cognitive approach for insomnia in psychiatric patients are scarce. One of the reference studies in the field includes a small number of bipolar patients, so we take caution in saying whether these techniques are useful for treatment of bipolar patients (Dashevsky and Kramer 1998). Nevertheless, although it is possible to treat bipolar insomnia with behavioral techniques, we think that this may not be the best choice because we have efficacious drugs to cope with it.

SUMMARY

Psychological treatments as add-ons to drugs may be appropriate for treating bipolar depression, but there is currently very little evidence indicating that such treatment is correct. What's more, not all bipolar depressions may respond to psychotherapy and we do not think that it should be a standard choice.

Our recommendation is to think of the inclusion of BCT or IPSRT in nonmelancholic depressions, particularly in those patients previously psychoeducated, and always as add-on to antidepressants or lamotrigine. Criteria for beginning psychotherapy with a certain patient should go beyond the mere existence of a psychosocial triggering factor or a personality disorder. In fact, these two criteria would be predictors of poor response to psychotherapy. Psychological interventions may successfully approach some nuclear depressive symptoms and might be included in treatment guidelines as soon as they show some efficacy in well-designed, randomized, clinical trials.

REFERENCES

American Psychiatric Association Steering Committee on Practice Guidelines: Treatment guidelines for bipolar disorder. Am J Psychiatry 159 (suppl 4):1–50, 2002

Blairy S, Linotte S, Souery D, et al: Social adjustment and self-esteem of bipolar patients: a multicentric study. J Affect Disord 79:97–103, 2004

Bowden CL, Krishnan AA: Pharmacotherapy for bipolar depression: an economic assessment. Expert Opin Pharmacother 5:1101–1107, 2004

Calabrese JR, Kasper S, Johnson G, et al: International consensus group on bipolar I depression treatment guidelines. J Clin Psychiatry 65:569–579, 2004

Colom F, Vieta E: Non-adherence in psychiatric disorders: misbehavior or clinical feature? Acta Psychiatr Scand 105:161–163, 2002a

Colom F, Vieta E: Treatment adherence in bipolar disorders. Clin Approaches Bipolar Disord 1:49–56, 2002b

Colom F, Vieta E, Martínez-Arán A, et al: A randomized trial on the efficacy of group psychoeducation in the prophylaxis of recurrences in bipolar patients whose disease is in remission. Arch Gen Psychiatry 60:402–407, 2003a

Colom F, Vieta E, Reinares M, et al: Psychoeducation efficacy in bipolar disorders beyond compliance enhancement. J Clin Psychiatry 4:1101–1105, 2003b

Dashevsky BA, Kramer M: Behavioral treatment of chronic insomnia in psychiatrically ill patients. J Clin Psychiatry 59:693–699, 1998

Elkin I, Shea MT, Watkins JT, et al: National Institute of Mental Health Treatment of Depression Collaborative Research Program: general effectiveness of treatments. Arch Gen Psychiatry 46:971–982, 1989

Elkin I, Gibbons R, Shea MT, et al: Initial severity and differential treatment outcome in the National Institute of Mental Health Ttreatment of Depression Collaborative Research Program. J Consult Clin Psychol 63:841–847, 1995

Frances AJ, Kahn DA, Carpenter D, et al: The expert consensus guidelines for treating depression in bipolar disorder. J Clin Psychiatry 59 (suppl 4):73–79, 1998

Frank E: Interpersonal and social rhythm therapy prevents depressive symptomatology in bipolar I patients. Bipolar Disord 1(suppl):13, 1999

Frank E, Kupfer DJ, Perel JM, et al: Three-year outcome for maintenance therapies in recurrent depression. Arch Gen Psychiatry 47:1093–1099, 1990

Frank E, Kupfer DJ, Wagner EF, et al: Efficacy of interpersonal psychotherapy as a maintenance treatment of recurrent depression: contributing factors. Arch Gen Psychiatry 48:1053–1059, 1991

Frank E, Swartz HA, Malinger AG, et al: Adjunctive psychotherapy for bipolar disorder: effects of changing treatment modality. J Abnor Psychol 108:579–587, 1999

Ghaemi SN, Hsu DJ, Soldani F, et al: Antidepressants in bipolar disorder: the case for caution. Bipolar Disord 5:421–433, 2003

Ghaemi SN, Rosenquist KJ, Ko JY, et al: Antidepressant treatment in bipolar versus unipolar depression. Am J Psychiatry 161:163–165, 2004

Giedke H, Schwarzler F: Therapeutic use of sleep deprivation in depression. Sleep Med Rev 6:361–377, 2002

Goodwin FK, Jamison KR: Manic-Depressive Illness. New York, Oxford University Press, 1990

Goodwin GM, Consensus Group of the British Association for Psychopharmacology: Evidence-based guidelines for treating recommendations from British Association for Psychopharmacology. J Psychopharmacol 17:149–173, 2003

Harrow M, Goldberg J, Grossman L, et al: Outcome in manic disorders: a naturalistic follow-up study. Arch Gen Psychiatry 47:665–671, 1990

Heim M: Effectiveness of bright light therapy in cyclothymic axis syndromes—a cross-over study in comparison with partial sleep deprivation. Psychiatr Neurol Med Psychol (Leipz) 40:269–277, 1988

Hirschfeld RM: Bipolar depression: the real challenge. Eur Neuropsychopharmacol 14 (suppl 2):83–88, 2004

Jacobs LI: Cognitive therapy of postmanic and postdepressive dysphoria in bipolar illness. Am J Psychother 36:450–458, 1982

Keller MB, McCullough JP, Klein DN, et al: A comparison of nefazodone, the cognitive behavioral-analysis system of psychotherapy, and their combination for the treatment of chronic depression. N Engl J Med 342:1462–1470, 2000

Klerman GL, Weissman MM, Rounsaville BJ, et al: Interpersonal Psychotherapy of Depression. New York, Basic Books, 1984

Lam DH, Watkins ER, Hayward P, et al: A randomized controlled study of cognitive therapy for relapse prevention for bipolar affective disorder. Outcome of the first year. Arch Gen Psychiatry 60:145–152, 2003

Lam D, Wright K, Smith N: Dysfunctional assumptions in bipolar disorder. J Affect Disord 79:193–199, 2004

Leahy RL, Beck AT: Cognitive therapy of depression and mania, in Depression and Mania. Edited by Gorgotas A, Cancro R. New York, Elsevier, 1988

Miklowitz DJ, Simoneau TL, George EL, et al: Family-focused treatment of bipolar disorder: 1-year effects of a psychoeducational program in conjunction with pharmacotherapy. Biol Psychiatry 48:582–592, 2000

Miklowitz DJ, George EL, Richards JA, et al: A randomized study of family focused psychoeducation and pharmacotherapy in the outpatient management of bipolar disorder. Arch Gen Psychiatry 60:904–912, 2003

Palmer A, Williams H, Adams M: CBT in a group format for bipolar affective disorder. Beh Cogn Psychother 23:153–168, 1995

Patelis-Siotis I, Young LT, Robb JC, et al: Group cognitive behavioral therapy for bipolar disorder: a feasibility and effectiveness study. J Affect Disord 65:145–153, 2001

Perry A, Tarrier N, Morris R, et al: Randomised controlled trial of efficacy of teaching patients with bipolar disorder to identify early symptoms of relapse and obtain treatment. Br Med J 318:149–153, 1999

Post RM, Leverich GS, Nolen WA, et al: A re-evaluation of the role of antidepressants in the treatment of bipolar depression: data from the Stanley Foundation Bipolar Network. Bipolar Disord 5:396–406, 2003

Rucci P, Frank E, Kostelnik B, et al: Suicide attempts in patients with bipolar I disorder during acute and maintenance phases of intensive treatment with pharmacotherapy and adjunctive psychotherapy. Am J Psychiatry 159:1160–1164, 2002

Schilgen B, Tolle R: Partial sleep deprivation as therapy for depression. Arch Gen Psychiatry 37:267–271, 1980

Scott J, Teasdale JD, Paykel ES, et al: Effects of cognitive therapy on psychological symptoms and social functioning in residual depression. Br J Psychiatry 177:440–446, 2000

Scott J, Garland A, Moorhead S: A pilot study of cognitive therapy in bipolar disorders. Psychol Med 31:459–467, 2001

Sharma V, Mazmanian DS, Persad E, et al: Treatment of bipolar depression: a survey of Canadian psychiatrists. Can J Psychiatry 42:298–302, 1997

Targum SD, Dibble ED, Davenport YB, et al: The Family Attitudes Questionnaire: Patients' and spouses' views of bipolar illness. Arch Gen Psychiatry 38:562–568, 1981

Vieta E: Case for caution, case for action. Bipolar Disord 5:434–435, 2003

Ward E, King M, Lloyd M, et al: Randomised controlled trial of non-directive counselling, cognitive-behaviour therapy, and usual general practitioner care for patients with depression. I: clinical effectiveness. Br Med J 321:1383–1388, 2000

Wehr TA: Can antidepressants induce rapid cycling? Arch Gen Psychiatry 50:495–496, 1993

Zaretsky A, Segal Z, Gemar M: Cognitive therapy for bipolar depression: a pilot study. Can J Psychiatry 44:491–494, 1999

11

FUTURE DIRECTIONS FOR PRACTICE AND RESEARCH

S. Nassir Ghaemi, M.D., M.P.H.
Jacclyn Saggese, B.A.
Frederick K. Goodwin, M.D.

UNTIL RELATIVELY RECENTLY, the development of new pharmacological treatments for depression focused so much on unipolar depression that *major depression* and *unipolar* seemed almost to be synonymous. Perhaps bipolar depression had taken a back seat because, until recently, all of the agents developed specifically for the treatment of bipolar disorder were introduced as antimanic agents. When depression did occur in a bipolar patient, it was treated with the same antidepressant agents developed for unipolar depression. Now, with the development of new agents (lamotrigine and perhaps also quetiapine) that may be more effective for bipolar than for unipolar depression, interest in bipolar depression has heightened. Another reason for this new emphasis on bipolar depression is recent longitudinal research indicating that depression represents the bulk of the morbidity associated with bipolar disorder. This component of the illness lasts much longer than the manic component, is harder to treat, and is associated with increased mortality. Depression is the core of bipolar illness.

Despite the advances of the past decade in practice and research, there is much room for progress. In this chapter, we will review a few directions in which future research and practice could go.

FROM CLINICAL PHENOMENOLOGY TO DIAGNOSTIC VALIDITY

The first subject that future research must clarify is the diagnostic validity of our current classification scheme. Considering just depression per se, are the bipolar and unipolar forms different? Unfortunately the structure of DSM-IV-TR distinguishes bipolar disorder as a separate illness distinct from all other mood disorders (i.e., from the depressive disorders). Thus, the current DSM system obscures the fact that, originally, the bipolar-unipolar distinction was conceived of as a way to distinguish two forms of a *recurrent* illness. In other words, the DSM structure gives precedence to polarity over cyclicity or recurrence, thereby obscuring the reality that one rather common variant of unipolar illness is as recurrent or cyclic, much like bipolar illness. Kraepelin's original focus on course and recurrence has been lost to the detriment of research and practice. Just as the wastebasket of disorders subsumed under the DSM-IV-TR diagnosis of unipolar major depressive disorder is too broad to be meaningful, the current definitions of bipolar disorder types I and II are probably too narrow. It remains for empirical research to demonstrate where the best line is to be drawn on the manic-depressive spectrum between these two varieties of depressive illness.

To accomplish this goal, validating methods need to be developed beyond their current state. For instance, more large-scale, community-based family studies, such as the Roscommon study (Kendler et al. 1993a), are much needed.

Validity studies also can be used to sharpen the reliability of diagnostic criteria for mood disorders. Such sharpening would have an impact on the current estimates of the prevalence of mood disorders, which are based substantially on the Epidemiological Catchment Area (ECA) study using the Diagnostic Interview Schedule (DIS) as its instrument (based on DSM-III) administered by lay persons. It is interesting to note, however, that clinician-administered research interviews correlated poorly with DIS-based diagnoses in one of the ECA sites (Anthony et al. 1985). Later, ECA-like diagnostic methods were used in the National Comorbidity Survey; even with similar methods, the prevalence of mania was twice as high as in the ECA study (1.6% compared with 0.8%) and the prevalence of unipolar depression was also much higher (17% vs. 8%) (Kessler et al. 1994). Rediagnosis of a subsample in that study by clinician researchers reported lower rates of nonaffective psychosis diagnoses than those made by trained lay interviewers (Kendler et al. 1996). Recent epidemiological studies have not improved upon or avoided these problems of diagnostic validity. For instance, large-scale applications of the self-report instrument, the Mood Disorder Questionnaire (MDQ), face the problem of low sensitivity and low positive predictive value in the community (Hirschfeld et al. 2003) or primary care (Das et al. 2005), as opposed to the clinical psychiatric setting (Hirschfeld et al. 2000). Future studies of such screening instruments need to emphasize, at least in the primary care setting, ways to combine such self-report scales with clinical clues to bipolar illness and input from family members, so as to improve the accuracy of bipolar diagnosis.

Clinicians do not always agree among themselves about mood disorder diagnoses either. For instance, in our research on diagnostic patterns in the community, we found that only 63% of patients who we diagnosed with bipolar disorder received that diagnosis from previous psychiatrists (Ghaemi et al. 2000). Similar misdiagnosis rates, about 50%, have been found using the MDQ in the clinical psychiatric setting (Hirschfeld et al. 2003). While some of this represents too much reliance on the depressed patient as the sole source of information (that is, a family member is not interviewed), part of this diagnostic disagreement may represent different interpretations of the available information. Future research needs to investigate factors involved with these reliability questions in mood disorders, and the implications for clinical and treatment studies. A relevant factor may be the phenomenon of lack of insight into the manic phase of bipolar disorder (Ghaemi and Rosenquist 2004), which can lead to misdiagnosis and, in addition to input from the family, may require sophisticated interviewing techniques that are difficult to standardize for research purposes.

PROGRESS IN NEUROBIOLOGY

There are a number of clinical features of bipolar depression that ought to be the focus of pathophysiological investigations (Goodwin and Jamison 1990): First, it appears that multiple central nervous system (CNS) functions play a role in the illness. Second, depressive episodes are often reactive to the environment. Third, there is a genetic vulnerability to affective illness. Fourth, there is a delayed onset of clinical symptoms, usually during the second or third decades of life. Fifth, spontaneous recovery occurs and episodes can be recurrent. Lastly, there is a lag in medication response time of usually 4–6 weeks after initial synaptic changes begin. This point is especially significant because the clinical pharmacology of therapeutic medications has served as one useful road map to testable biological hypotheses ("the pharmacological bridge").

It is our view that the ideal neurobiological hypothesis must explain the two most fundamental features of mood disorders: genetic vulnerability and episodic recurrence. In this regard, most biological studies of patients involve the illness state, whereas many studies of potential biological markers (especially in clinical genetic studies) involve the recovered states. If one wishes to truly identify trait markers of biological predisposition, it is imperative to study subjects prior to the onset of the illness. Such trials may be possible in longitudinal investigation of at-risk populations.

The state-trait differentiation is, in any case, an important distinction that needs to be made to avoid confusing and conflicting reports. Neuroendocrine changes, such as increased corticosteroid activity, may be present during the illness state but not in the premorbid or recovered states. Furthermore, premorbid pathological processes may differ from illness state–related processes as well as from trait markers during later recovered phases. Research in children and adolescents who are at risk before the onset of illness also may assist in uncovering the pathogenesis of affective illness. Such work may help clarify which neurobiological findings may represent etiological processes and which ones may represent normal homeostatic mechanisms, perhaps with only secondary pathologic effects (Post 1992).

Advances in neuroimaging are another exciting area of progress in neurobiological research. Mood disorders still lag behind schizophrenia in being a focus of such work, and future neuroimaging research should focus more on mood disorders. The relative paucity of work in mood disorders raises the likelihood of type II error (false negatives) in the interpretation of available small data sets due to lack of statistical power to find existent differences. Functional neuroimaging, like positron emission tomography (PET), is beginning to demonstrate subtle pathophysiological differences that have eluded structural brain imaging, such as computed tomography (CT) or magnetic resonance imaging (MRI) (Mayberg 2003). Recent data suggest neuroanatomical mechanisms of antidepressant response in unipolar depression (Mayberg et al. 2005); similar work needs to be done in bipolar depression.

Two lines of investigation that relate directly to the unique clinical feature of recurrence in mood disorders also should have increased emphasis in future research. The first posits that clinical recurrence involves abnormalities in biological rhythms, especially circadian cycles, an area pioneered by Wehr and his colleagues (1983). The second draws an analogy between the episodic nature of mood disorders and electrical kindling, with behavioral sensitization to mood episodes, a hypothesis developed most extensively by Post and associates (1992).

Research on circadian rhythms suggests that abnormalities involving the suprachiasmatic nuclei (SCN) in the hypothalamus may explain many of the clinical features of recurrent mood disorders (including seasonality of episode type) through secondary effects on neurotransmitter systems. Free-running rhythms, cycles that are not entrained to the 24-hour day-night cycle, may desynchronize other circadian rhythms, thereby adversely affecting mood (Wehr and Goodwin 1983). This hypothesis recently has been supported by an animal model of a genetically fast biological clock in rats missing the tau gene, with behavioral characteristics roughly analogous to bipolar symptoms. Future directions for research on biological clocks should seek to identify potential abnormalities in patients with mood disorders in general and seasonal affective disorder in particular. Eventually, the genetic differences behind abnormal clocks may be identified, which can lead to an understanding of the proteins translated by those genes and thereby clarify specific pathophysiological mechanisms of mood disorder.

The second hypothesis relevant to recurrence is the kindling paradigm. As advanced by Post and his associates (1992), this theory builds on the physiological finding that intermittent, subthreshold electrical or chemical stimuli will produce increasingly strong neuronal depolarization in the limbic system; such depolarization can lead to an independent permanent seizure focus, with possible behavioral effects similar to mood disorders. While a direct link between kindling phenomena and clinical recurrence cannot readily be established, the hypothesis does possess the advantage of explaining a number of clinical findings in one theory: first, earlier episodes of bipolar disorder tend to be precipitated by environmental stressors, whereas later episodes tend to be triggered less often psychosocially; second, the severity of untreated mood episodes tends to worsen over time; third, the interval between mood episodes decreases over time; and fourth, stressful childhood events may predispose one to mood disorders in adulthood (Kendler et al. 1992). This last feature is particularly supported by animal data that suggest that younger animals are more sensitive to kindling at lower levels of intensity than older animals (Fanelli and McNamara 1986). This raises the possibility of early preventative pharmacological (antikindling) treatment once genetic markers are identified.

DIRECTIONS FOR GENETIC RESEARCH

Twin studies are beginning to provide guidance not only to the genetic components of illness but to the environmental factors that might be relevant. In one study, liability to major depression or generalized anxiety disorder was explained by a genetic model involving a large contribution of additive, nonmendelian genetic inheritance and a smaller contribution of specific environmental effects ("the slings and arrows of outrageous fortune"); no significant contribution could be found for either mendelian genetic inheritance (i.e., dominant or recessive qualitative patterns, as opposed to additive quantitative patterns) or for shared (i.e., family) environmental effects (Kendler et al. 1993b). This result would suggest that psychosocial research should concentrate on current environmental stressors rather than childhood or family experiences, as has traditionally been the case. Further work is needed to confirm or refute these suggestive findings.

To expand on this theme, one of the most consistently observed associations between early psychosocial factors and the development of mental disorders in adults has been the correlation between childhood parental loss and major depression. To our knowledge, the only study of this relationship that has used a genetically informative sample is that of Kendler et al. (1992), who extensively studied a large cohort of female twins ($N=1,030$), 57% of whom were monozygotic. After factoring out genetic contributions and using multiple regression and relative risk analyses, this group found evidence for a modest effect of either parental separation or death or both on the risk of major depression, generalized anxiety disorder, and panic disorder or phobia in the offspring. However, the percentage of the total variance in liability due to nongenetic factors operating earlier in childhood was small, ranging from 1.6% to 4.9%. For major depression in these adults, the genetic contribution was approximately 25 times more important than the early psychological impact of parental loss in childhood. Nevertheless, when recent stressful events were considered, their presence was the single most powerful predictor of major depression. Due to this importance of current or recent stress in precipitating episodes, Kendler and colleagues were able to conclude that genetics plays a substantial but not overwhelming role in influencing the onset of depression.

Eventually, work on the genetic and environmental susceptibilities to mood disorder should be linked with the development of neurobiological changes in the course of the illness. We should then be able to understand why certain treatments work and others do not, and we should be able to tailor treatments more specifically to the mood disorder at hand based on its etiological roots and neurobiological mechanisms. Recent work has begun to look at pharmacogenetic predictors of response or side effects. For instance, the serotonin transporter gene polymorphism (Rousseva et al. 2003) and catechol O-methyltransferase hypoactivity (Papolos et al. 1998) have been linked to antidepressant-induced mania or ultra–rapid cycling, respectively.

ADVANCES IN CLINICAL PSYCHOPHARMACOLOGY

Without doubt, the greatest practical advance in the treatment of bipolar depression has been the development of lamotrigine as a mood stabilizer with a prominent long-term benefit for depressive symptoms (Calabrese et al. 2003). Despite its small, but real, risk for Stevens-Johnson syndrome, lamotrigine is also generally well tolerated, thus providing patients an alternative to other mood stabilizers (which have only modest effects against depression and substantially more side effects) and antidepressants (which carry some risk of long-term destabilization in addition to more side effects).

Nevertheless, many patients still do not respond to or do not tolerate lamotrigine. Unfortunately, the last decade has not seen much progress in knowledge about the efficacy and safety of traditional antidepressants in bipolar depression. As reviewed in a recent meta-analysis (Gijsman et al. 2004), only five placebo-controlled, randomized clinical trials (RCTs) of antidepressants seem to exist, and only two have occurred in the last decade (the other three took place in the 1980s and involved seligiline or fluoxetine mostly in the absence of mood stabilizers). Of the two newer studies, one (Tohen et al. 2003) was a huge study (N=833) of olanzapine compared with olanzapine plus fluoxetine (OFC) or placebo; this was the largest study ever conducted on bipolar depression. Unfortunately, with such a huge sample, a clinically trivial benefit with olanzapine alone was statistically significant, leading to some confusion about whether this agent is effective in bipolar depression. The benefit of OFC was more noticeable and led to the only current U.S. Federal Drug Administration indication of any treatment for acute bipolar depression. However, this benefit has not yet been shown to continue into long-term treatment, and it is not even clear if the olanzapine part of that combination is conferring any benefit beyond antimanic protection. The other antidepressant study in recent years is perhaps the only truly well-designed and clinically meaningful study—the comparison of paroxetine versus imipramine versus placebo, added to lithium (Nemeroff et al. 2001). That study found lithium alone at therapeutic levels (>0.8) as effective as the addition of antidepressants.

In sum, we still do not possess a single well-designed study that proves efficacy of any antidepressant, even acutely, for bipolar depression, when compared with proven mood stabilizers like lithium, which is why more antidepressant studies are desperately needed in bipolar disorder research.

Will atypical antipsychotics prove helpful for bipolar depression? The olanzapine data, described above, are rather equivocal. However, a recent study has found benefit with quetiapine in bipolar depression, with a much larger effect size and more benefit for core mood symptoms (as opposed to neurovegetative symptoms) than the above olanzapine study (Calabrese et al. 2005). Such benefit may represent antidepressant efficacy, or it may represent improvement in persons with mixed mood states subthreshold for strict DSM-IV-TR mixed episode criteria. Further replication will be needed to clarify this apparent benefit with quetiapine in bipolar depression.

The nature and frequency of acute manic switch, as well as long-term destabilization, with antidepressants in bipolar depression also needs to be established by larger studies and better designed, large epidemiological studies.

Future clinical trial designs would also benefit from randomized crossover of treatment nonresponders, as well as an emphasis on clinical and neurobiological factors that predict response. Such work would allow future investigators to target specific antidepressant agents to patients with certain clinical or neurobiological features and would allow systematic decision making in the course of switching among antidepressant agents.

Beyond the short-term efficacy and safety of antidepressants, the controversy about their long-term risks has intensified. Observational studies now are being published on both sides of the divide, some suggesting that antidepressants make some patients with bipolar disorder worse in the long run (Ghaemi et al. 2003), while others suggest that antidepressants lead to good outcomes (Altshuler et al. 2003). In order for clinicians to come to a consensus, we must increase the RCTs of the maintenance efficacy and safety of new antidepressants in bipolar depression. New studies (Ghaemi et al. 2005; Post et al. 2004) are nearing completion and will provide some guidance to clinicians in the future, but larger replications will be needed.

It is imperative that we obtain such data because this is a major public health problem. If we find out that antidepressants are indeed ineffective in most patients and harmful in an appreciable number, it would then mean that clinicians have been unnecessarily exposing the patient population to such agents for decades. It is crucial that this matter be clarified and that clinical practice be altered drastically within the next decade.

INTEGRATING BIOLOGICAL AND PSYCHOSOCIAL ASPECTS OF MOOD DISORDER

Future conceptualizations of mood disorder are less likely to suffer from the reductionistic effects of Cartesian dualism than they did in the past. Given the emerging realization that mind and brain are not different entities belonging to different realms of experience, the distinction between the biological and the psychosocial aspects of illness begins to break down. This approach is supported by advances in biological research itself. New developments in neuroscience are beginning to show that even subtle changes in the environment (especially early in life) can result in long-lasting changes in the brain. These advances are based on new insights into the plasticity of the CNS, with elegant demonstrations of often-specific environmental influences on specific neurobiological processes, including gene expression. In the study of stress effects, for example, the field has moved rapidly beyond the immediate, often short-term biological responses (e.g., hypothalamic-pituitary-adrenal axis activation) to demonstrations of environmental manipulations producing long-lasting, even permanent, changes (Gynther et al. 1998). These changes have been shown to operate through receptor-coupled, intracellular, signal transduction pathways regulating gene expression that, in turn, alters the syntheses of specific proteins and cell components (Manji 1992). Kandel has suggested that a mechanism of action for psychotherapy may involve alterations in synaptic structure and function (Kandel 1999). If this is true, then medication treatment and psychotherapy may be acting through a similar final common pathway of altered brain function. This possibility is supported by work in obsessive-compulsive disorder (Baer 1996), in which cognitive-behavior therapy (CBT) produced similar changes in PET neuroimaging, as did antidepressant treatment with serotonin reuptake inhibitors. Interestingly, in a study of 30 unipolar depressed outpatients (Goldapple et al. 2004), those who responded to CBT had a different pattern of PET changes (prefrontal decreases in activity and hippocampal/cingulate increases) than those who responded to paroxetine (prefrontal increases in activity and hippocampal/cingulate decreases). More work will be needed in this fruitful field of translating psychotherapeutic treatment into alterations in brain structure and function.

Once the brain is understood to be the final common pathway for both medication and psychotherapy treatments, then the conflict between biological and psychosocial approaches becomes more manageable. Both treatment approaches are mediated by the brain. It may be that mood disorders may have largely biological origins and yet are responsive to psychotherapy. Conversely, some forms of mood disorder may be largely psychosocial in origin, and yet respond to medication treatment. It is an elementary error of logic to reason from conclusion to premises; one must always work the other way around. Hence, although the efficacy of pharmacological or psychotherapeutic treatments may give us clues about where we need to look in the search for the etiologies of mood disorders, the fact that these treatments may work in themselves does not establish any specific etiology.

Certainly, an important goal is to integrate psychopharmacological clinical trials with psychotherapeutic aims of treatment and to include combinations of the two treatment modalities as well. This research has valuable practical implications; for instance, current data suggest that decisions regarding medication as a component of treatment versus psychotherapy alone (specifically, interpersonal or cognitive-behavioral therapy) should be based more on the nature of the symptoms and especially on whether an illness is recurrent or not, than on speculative etiological bases for the illness. The latter point regarding recurrence is reinforced by Frank et al.'s (1990) landmark study comparing imipramine, interpersonal therapy, a combination of the two, and placebo, in which those with three or more episodes responded better to medication or combination treatment than to psychotherapy alone. In other studies of patients with one or two episodes of illness, CBT tended to be as effective as medication treatment for acute mild to moderate depression (Elkin et al. 1989). In bipolar disorder, a number of recent studies are showing more benefits with psychotherapies (such as group psychoeducation or family-focused therapies) (Colom et al. 2003; Miklowitz and Craighead 2001) than seen with many medications, such as antidepressants, in similar designs (Ghaemi et al. 2001). Recent clinical trials sponsored by the pharmaceutical industry have begun to follow the lead established by pioneering work on combined psychotherapy and medication treatment studies sponsored by the National Institute of Mental Health in previous decades. We hope this trend will continue.

QUALITY OF LIFE AND FUNCTIONAL IMPAIRMENT

We must no longer limit ourselves to evaluating treatments by focusing on symptoms alone. In unipolar depression research and practice, the die has been cast. Treatment response, defined as 50% or more improvement in mood symptoms, is no longer sufficient. Remission—the near complete removal of depressive symptoms—is the goal (Thase et al. 2002) because it has been shown that even mild to moderate residual symptoms are associated with continued functional impairment in patients with unipolar depressive illness (Thase 2001). Similar observations have been made with bipolar disorder (Altshuler et al. 2002). Furthermore, it has been shown that symptomatic improvement in bipolar disorder does not lead to functional improvement in all cases. In one study, despite syndromal recovery, about 40% of patients who had recovered from an initial manic episode had not achieved functional recovery (Tohen et al. 2000). Some of the continued functional impairment, even in patients with bipolar disorder who achieve euthymia, may have to do with long-term cognitive impairment (Martinez-Aran et al. 2004; van Gorp et al. 1998). Such cognitive impairment may be the consequence of excitotoxic effects of catecholamine overactivity during repeated mood episodes (Altshuler 1993; Lampe et al. 2003). Addressing cognitive impairment in persons with bipolar disorder will be an important task for researchers and clinicians. The new generation of cognitive enhancing agents may have potential in this regard.

Nevertheless, it is not entirely clear that our medications will bring us to the goal of remission. As noted above, the use of psychotherapies together with medications have not been tried with sufficient vigor. Medications are often blunt instruments in bipolar disorder, overshooting or undershooting the mark of euthymia: when one tries to achieve remission by using several medications in combination, the likelihood of increased side effects that can undermine functioning and quality of life must be carefully weighed; one should also pay careful attention to the potential of psychotherapy to improve overall functioning. Therefore, future clinical trials should focus on quality of life and functional impairment as key outcomes, and clinicians should focus on such issues, and not just symptom status, as they choose among treatments. This approach may lead to the use of fewer rather than more medications as the balance of side effects and benefits is weighed—at least until more tolerable effective medications are developed for bipolar disorder.

ETHICS AND PUBLIC POLICY: NEW QUESTIONS

The ability to conduct research and adequately advance knowledge in mood disorders is dependent to a great degree on government-sponsored funds. While working with families and patient advocacy groups, the profession needs to be more involved in communicating with and participating in governmental structures to ensure that such funding is available. As the federal budget is tightened in the United States, research funding is increasingly found in the private sector, mainly in the pharmaceutical industry. For investigators participating in pharmaceutical industry–sponsored research, it is necessary not only to appreciate the benefits that accrue for both the industry and society from advances in this research, but also to recognize that the private sector may have financial interests that may not be shared by society at large. The recent debate about antidepressants and risk of suicide (Cipriani et al. 2005) has brought this issue to the forefront. As scientists, future researchers will have to continue to promote the needs of science and society as primary, while also acknowledging that much less research would be possible without the involvement of the pharmaceutical industry. Hopefully, psychotherapy research can be integrated into these efforts.

There is also a potential negative impact of ethical constraints on the ability to adequately conduct scientific studies. In some placebo-controlled studies of bipolar disorder, more severely ill patients are often excluded by clinicians who are rightfully concerned about the risks of such nontreatment. However, as a consequence, we often see relatively small effect sizes for the difference between drug and placebo in the less severely ill patients who enter those studies. Sometimes these small effect sizes are seized upon by critics as evidence of lack of benefit with psychotropic medications. This kind of rationale has been used with antidepressants, both in children and adults, and with some mood stabilizers, such as the divalproex prophylaxis study. Our profession needs to reach a better consensus about how to achieve ethical protections while at the same time being able to study severely ill patients in randomized clinical trials.

Another area of concern is the impact of managed care on innovation. As academic centers become more constricted by managed care insurance reimbursement, little is left of the funds previously used to support the salaries of researchers who conducted unfunded or institutionally funded research. Where the delayed benefits of research discoveries are sacrificed for the immediate benefit of cost containment, legitimate concerns arise. A more subtle but, in the long run, more serious concern arises from the transformation of guidelines into recipes. Historically, innovation in medicine has often started with a clinician trying something unconventional. These initial unsystematic observations are then subjected to study by the research community, eventually separating the wheat from the chaff. But if rigid guidelines become a disincentive to innovation, long-term progress in the future will be seriously threatened.

SUMMARY

The future of practice and research in bipolar depression is dependent on a number of scientific and political factors. Although advances have been made in the last decade, the state of our knowledge about bipolar depression is still markedly limited, especially when compared with our knowledge of unipolar depression. We need more diagnostic work to clarify the boundaries of bipolar depression, more neurobiological and genetic work on predictors of response, more serious work on psychotherapies, and a new focus on quality of life and functional impairment. In the process, we need to pay attention to political and economic trends that have hampered such processes—especially shrinking government funding of clinical research, unnecessarily stringent ethical constraints, and the harmful impact of managed care on academic centers. The two-edged influence of the pharmaceutical industry (as a major sponsor of clinical research—but with a private agenda) also needs to be acknowledged honestly and straightforwardly, and managed with the interests of the public first and foremost.

Clinicians and researchers face a future that could go in many directions. Hopefully the directions taken will lead to further advances in understanding and treating this important illness.

REFERENCES

Altshuler LL: Bipolar disorder: are repeated episodes associated with neuroanatomic and cognitive changes? Biol Psychiatry 33:563–565, 1993

Altshuler LL, Gitlin MJ, Mintz J, et al: Subsyndromal depression is associated with functional impairment in patients with bipolar disorder. J Clin Psychiatry 63:807–811, 2002

Altshuler L, Suppes T, Black D, et al: Impact of antidepressant discontinuation after acute bipolar depression remission on rates of depressive relapse at 1-year follow-up. Am J Psychiatry 160:1252–1262, 2003

Anthony JC, Folstein M, Romanoski AJ: Comparison of lay DIS and a standardized psychiatric diagnosis. Arch Gen Psychiatry 42:667–675, 1985

Baer L: Behavior therapy: endogenous serotonin therapy? J Clin Psychiatry 57 (suppl 6):33–35, 1996

Calabrese J, Bowden C, Sachs G, et al: A placebo-controlled 18-month trial of lamotrigine and lithium maintenance treatment in recently depressed patients with bipolar I disorder. J Clin Psychiatry 64:1013–1024, 2003

Calabrese JR, Keck PE Jr, MacFadden W, et al: A randomized, double-blind, placebo-controlled trial of quetiapine in the treatment of bipolar I or II depression. Am J Psychiatry 162:1351–1360, 2005

Cipriani A, Barbui C, Geddes JR: Suicide, depression, and antidepressants. Br Med J 330:373–374, 2005

Colom F, Vieta E, Martinez-Aran A, et al: A randomized trial on the efficacy of group psychoeducation in the prophylaxis of recurrences in bipolar patients whose disease is in remission. Arch Gen Psychiatry 60:402–407, 2003

Das AK, Olfson M, Gameroff MJ, et al: Screening for bipolar disorder in a primary care practice. J Am Med Assoc 293:956–963, 2005

Elkin I, Shea MT, Watkins JT, et al: National Institute of Mental Health Treatment of Depression Collaborative Research Program: general effectiveness of treatments. Arch Gen Psychiatry 46:971–982, 1989

Fanelli RJ, McNamara JO: Effects of age on kindling and kindled seizure-induced increase of benzodiazepine receptor binding. Brain Res 362:17–22, 1986

Frank E, Kupfer DJ, Perel JM, et al: Three-year outcomes for maintenance therapies in recurrent depression. Arch Gen Psychiatry 47:1093–1099, 1990

Ghaemi SN, Rosenquist KJ: Is insight in mania state-dependent? A meta-analysis. J Nerv Ment Dis 192:771–775, 2004

Ghaemi SN, Boiman EE, Goodwin FK: Diagnosing bipolar disorder and the effect of antidepressants: a naturalistic study. J Clin Psychiatry 61:804–808, 2000

Ghaemi SN, Lenox MS, Baldessarini RJ: Effectiveness and safety of long-term antidepressant treatment in bipolar disorder. J Clin Psychiatry 62:565–569, 2001

Ghaemi SN, Hsu DJ, Soldani F, et al: Antidepressants in bipolar disorder: the case for caution. Bipolar Disord 5:421–433, 2003

Ghaemi SN, El-Mallakh RS, Baldassano CF, et al: A randomized clinical trial of efficacy and safety of long-term antidepressant use in bipolar disorder (abstract). Bipolar Disord 7 (suppl 2): 59, 2005

Gijsman HJ, Geddes JR, Rendell JM, et al: Antidepressants for bipolar depression: a systematic review of randomized, controlled trials. Am J Psychiatry 161:1537–1547, 2004

Goldapple K, Segal Z, Garson C, et al: Modulation of cortical-limbic pathways in major depression: treatment-specific effects of cognitive behavior therapy. Arch Gen Psychiatry 61:34–41, 2004

Goodwin FK, Jamison KR: Manic Depressive Illness. New York, Oxford University Press, 1990

Gynther BD, Calford MB, Sah P: Neuroplasticity and psychiatry. Aust N Z J Psychiatry 32:119–128, 1998

Hirschfeld RM, Williams JB, Spitzer RL, et al: Development and validation of a screening instrument for bipolar spectrum disorder: the Mood Disorder Questionnaire. Am J Psychiatry 157:1873–1875, 2000

Hirschfeld, RM, Calabrese JR, Weissman MM, et al: Screening for bipolar disorder in the community. J Clin Psychiatry 64:53–59, 2003

Kandel ER: Biology and the future of psychoanalysis: a new intellectual framework for psychiatry revisited. Am J Psychiatry 156:505–524, 1999

Kendler KS, Neale MC, Kessler RC, et al: Childhood parental loss and adult psychopathology in women. A twin study perspective. Arch Gen Psychiatry 49:109–116, 1992

Kendler KS, McGuire M, Gruenberg AM: The Roscommon family study, I: methods, diagnosis of probands, and risk of schizophrenia in relatives. Arch Gen Psychiatry 50:527–540, 1993a

Kendler KS, Walters EE, Neale MC: The structure of the genetic and environmental risk factors for six major psychiatric disorders in women. Arch Gen Psychiatry 52:374–383, 1993b

Kendler KS, Gallagher TJ, Abelson JM, et al: Lifetime prevalence, demographic risk factors, and diagnostic validity of nonaffective psychosis as assessed in a US community sample: the national comorbidity survey. Arch Gen Psychiatry 53:1022–1031, 1996

Kessler RC, McGonagle KA, Zhao S: Lifetime and 12-month prevalence of DSM-III-R psychiatric disorders in the United States. Arch Gen Psychiatry 51:8–19, 1994

Lampe IK, Hulshoff Pol HE, Janssen J, et al: Association of depression duration with reduction of global cerebral gray matter volume in female patients with recurrent major depressive disorder. Am J Psychiatry 160:2052–2054, 2003

Manji HK: G proteins: implications for psychiatry. Am J Psychiatry 149:746–760, 1992

Martinez-Aran A, Vieta E, Colom F, et al: Cognitive impairment in euthymic bipolar patients: implications for clinical and functional outcome. Bipolar Disord 6:224–232, 2004

Mayberg HS: Positron emission tomography imaging in depression: a neural systems perspective. Neuroimaging Clin N Am 13:805–815, 2003

Mayberg HS, Lozano AM, Voon V, et al: Deep brain stimulation for treatment-resistant depression. Neuron 45:651–660, 2005

Miklowitz D, Craighead W: Bipolar affective disorder: does psychosocial treatment add to the efficacy of drug therapy? Economics of Neuroscience 3:58–64, 2001

Nemeroff CB, Evans DL, Gyulai L, et al: Double-blind, placebo-controlled comparison of imipramine and paroxetine in the treatment of bipolar depression. Am J Psychiatry 158:906–912, 2001

Papolos DF, Veit S, Faedda GL, et al: Ultra-ultra rapid cycling bipolar disorder is associated with the low activity catecholamine-O-methyltransferase allele. Mol Psychiatry 3:346–349, 1998

Post RM: The transduction of psychosocial stress into the neurobiology of recurrent affective illness. Am J Psychiatry 149:999–1010, 1992

Post R, Altshuler L, Leverich G, et al: Randomized comparison of bupropion, sertraline, and venlafaxine as adjunctive treatment in acute bipolar depression, in Program and Abstracts, American Psychiatric Association 157th Annual Meeting, New York, May 1–6, 2004. Washington, DC, American Psychiatric Association, 2004, pp 259–265

Rousseva A, Henry C, van den Bulke D, et al: Antidepressant-induced mania, rapid cycling and the serotonin transporter gene polymorphism. Pharmacogenomics J 3:101–104, 2003

Thase ME: The clinical, psychosocial, and pharmacoeconomic ramifications of remission. Am J Manag Care 7:S377–S385, 2001

Thase ME, Sloan DM, Kornstein SG: Remission as the critical outcome of depression treatment. Psychopharmacol Bull 36:12–25, 2002

Tohen M, Hennen J, Zarate CJ, et al: The McLean first episode project: two-year syndromal and functional recovery in 219 cases of major affective disorders with psychotic features. Am J Psychiatry 157:220–228, 2000

Tohen M, Vieta E, Calabrese J, et al: Efficacy of olanzapine and olanzapine-fluoxetine combination in the treatment of bipolar I depression. Arch Gen Psychiatry 60:1079–1088, 2003

van Gorp WG, Altshuler L, Theberge DC, et al: Cognitive impairment in euthymic bipolar patients with and without prior alcohol dependence. A preliminary study. Arch Gen Psychiatry 55:41–46, 1998

Wehr TA, Goodwin FK: Biological rhythms in manic-depressive illness, in Circadian Rhythms in Psychiatry. Edited by Wehr TA, Goodwin FK. Pacific Grove, CA, Boxwood Press, 1983, pp 129–184

Index

*Page numbers printed in **boldface** type refer to tables or figures.*